The Peptide Bioregulator Revolution

A Comprehensive Guide to Anti-Aging, Performance Enhancement, and Optimal Health for Youthful Vitality, Muscle Growth, and Brain Boost

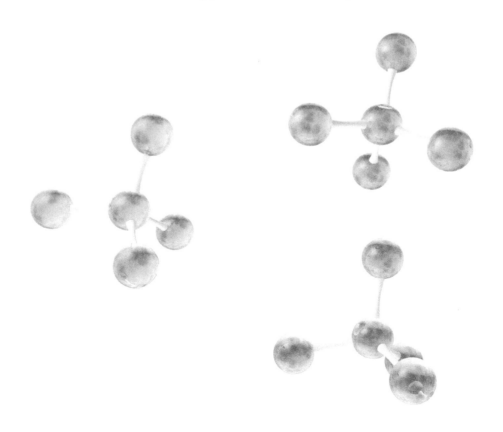

Matthew Clarke-Hunter

Table of Contents

INTRODUCTION

H ave you ever wondered if there's a natural way to slow down the aging process or boost your mental clarity? Enter the realm of peptide bioregulators—a groundbreaking class of molecules that could be the key to unlocking your true potential. In an age where wellness is more than just a trend, it's a lifestyle, these tiny but mighty molecules are making waves in the health and fitness community.

Today, we live in a society obsessed with wellness, always searching for shortcuts and quick fixes to better health. From synthetic supplements to invasive surgeries, the avenues explored to achieve optimal health can be endless and sometimes overwhelming. However, within this storm of options, peptide bioregulators stand out like a beacon, promising not only scientifically backed results but also a natural approach to enhancing life quality. Isn't it time we turn to nature for solutions?

Take a moment to imagine improving your skin's elasticity and vitality, naturally boosting your athletic performance, or even enhancing your cognitive functions without relying on artificial means. Peptide bioregulators offer all these benefits and more. They are transforming our understanding of health, promising not just better aging, but a better life overall.

In this book, you'll embark on a journey through the fascinating world of peptide bioregulators. We'll dive into what they are, how they work, and why they might just be the natural solution you've been searching for. To guide you effectively, the book is structured across fifteen chapters, each designed to unveil the science, applications, and practical ways to incorporate these powerful molecules into your daily routine.

We'll start by exploring the basics—what peptide bioregulators are and how they were discovered. From there, we'll move into the science behind these molecules, delving into their mechanisms of action and why they are so effective. Each chapter will build on the last, providing a comprehensive understanding and actionable insights.

For those particularly interested in anti-aging solutions, we have dedicated sections that explain how peptide bioregulators can help promote youthful skin, improve bone density, and support overall longevity. Imagine reducing wrinkles and fine lines naturally, without the need for expensive creams or painful injections.

Athletes and fitness aficionados will find immense value in the portions of the book focused on performance enhancement. We'll discuss how peptide bioregulators can assist in muscle growth, expedite recovery times, and increase stamina. Picture yourself running faster, lifting heavier weights, and recovering quicker—all thanks to the power of these natural molecules.

Busy professionals who are constantly juggling multiple tasks will benefit from our deep dive into cognitive health. Learn about how peptide bioregulators can enhance focus, memory, and mental clarity, helping you stay sharp and productive throughout your hectic day. Whether you're preparing for a big presentation or simply trying to keep up with the demands of modern life, these insights can make a significant difference in your performance and well-being.

Finally, for those who lean towards holistic health approaches, including alternative medicine and wellness supplements, the later chapters will resonate deeply. Discover how peptide bioregulators fit into a broader scheme of natural health practices, complementing other methods you may already be using.

Throughout these chapters, we'll also share inspiring real-life stories and testimonials from individuals who have experienced transformative changes thanks to peptide bioregulators. These narratives will not only motivate you but also provide practical examples of how you can integrate peptide bioregulators into your life.

Moreover, we'll include expert opinions and scientific studies that back up the claims made, ensuring you have access to credible information. The goal here is not just to inform but to empower you with knowledge so you can make informed decisions about your health.

By the end of this book, you will have a thorough understanding of peptide bioregulators and the myriad ways they can enhance your life. Whether you are looking to slow down the aging process, boost your mental clarity, improve your athletic performance, or simply incorporate more natural solutions into your health regimen, this book will serve as your ultimate guide.

Ready to explore a new dimension of health and wellness? Let's embark on this enlightening journey together, discovering how peptide bioregulators can help you unlock your true potential for a healthier, happier, and longer life.

CHAPTER 1

Introduction to Peptide Bioregulators

P eptide bioregulators are short chains of amino acids essential for regulating various biological functions within the human body. These naturally occurring compounds operate differently from traditional pharmaceuticals and supplements, targeting fundamental cellular processes instead of specific symptoms or diseases. Their unique approach allows them to influence gene expression, protein synthesis, and enzymatic activity, providing a holistic mechanism for maintaining health and promoting wellness. By understanding the role of peptide bioregulators in bodily functions, we can appreciate their potential benefits in various health contexts, from enhancing athletic performance to addressing age-related conditions.

In this chapter, we will delve into the definition and historical background of peptide bioregulators, exploring how their discovery has shaped modern health practices. We will examine the differences between peptide bioregulators and traditional pharmaceuticals, highlighting the advantages of using peptides in health management. The chapter will also cover significant milestones and researchers who have contributed to our understanding of peptides, illustrating how these small molecules have transformed medical and wellness fields. Furthermore, we will discuss current trends and research focusing on new peptide applications, emphasizing the ongoing evolution and future potential of peptide bioregulators in diverse health and wellness strategies.

Definition and History

Peptide bioregulators are short chains of amino acids that serve as crucial agents in regulating various biological functions within our bodies. Unlike traditional pharmaceuticals, which often target specific symptoms or diseases, peptide bioregulators work at a more fundamental level. They assist in the regulation of cellular processes and communication, ensuring that bodily systems operate efficiently. For instance, these bioregulators can influence gene expression, protein synthesis, and enzymatic activity. This comprehensive approach allows peptide bioregulators to affect multiple aspects of health, making them unique compared to traditional treatments.

Traditional pharmaceuticals and supplements typically offer targeted solutions aimed at treating specific conditions or deficiencies. Pharmaceuticals often come with a range of side effects due to their synthetic nature and focused action on particular pathways. Supplements, on the other hand, generally provide nutrients that may assist in wellness but often lack a targeted mechanism of action. In contrast, peptide bioregulators are naturally occurring compounds that seamlessly integrate with the body's existing systems. Their ability to modulate biological functions without causing significant side effects sets them apart from conventional medical and dietary interventions.

Understanding the historical context of peptide bioregulators is essential to appreciate their role in modern health practices. The discovery of peptide bioregulators dates back to the early 20th century when scientists first started to isolate and understand these compounds. Initial research focused on identifying various peptides and understanding their roles in physiological processes. Over time, advancements in biochemistry and molecular biology accelerated the pace of discoveries, leading to a deeper understanding of how peptide bioregulators function.

One of the landmark moments in peptide research was the isolation of insulin in the 1920s. Insulin, a peptide hormone, revolutionized the treatment of diabetes and showcased the potential of peptides in medical applications. Following this discovery, researchers around the world began exploring other peptides, uncovering their roles in growth, metabolism, and immune response. The 20th century saw numerous key studies that highlighted the importance of peptides in maintaining health and promoting healing.

Several key researchers have made significant contributions to the field of peptide bioregulators. Dr. Frederick Banting and Charles Best's discovery of insulin laid the groundwork for future peptide research. In the mid-20th century, researchers like Roger Guillemin and Andrew Schally further expanded the understanding of peptides by discovering hypothalamic hormones, earning them the Nobel Prize in Physiology or Medicine in 1977. Their work demonstrated how peptides could regulate complex hormonal systems, paving the way for new therapeutic possibilities.

In recent decades, the study of peptide bioregulators has continued to evolve, driven by technological advancements and an increasing interest in natural and holistic approaches to health. Modern research focuses on identifying new peptides and understanding their mechanisms of action. This ongoing exploration has revealed the diverse roles of peptides in areas such as neuroprotection, tissue regeneration, and immune modulation. As a result, peptide bioregulators are now being investigated for their potential to treat a wide range of conditions, from age-related diseases to cognitive decline.

The growing body of evidence supporting the efficacy of peptide bioregulators has prompted their inclusion in various health and wellness strategies. For example, athletes and fitness enthusiasts leverage peptides for muscle growth, performance enhancement, and faster recovery times. These compounds help optimize physiological functions, allowing individuals to achieve their fitness goals more effectively. Additionally, busy professionals concerned about cognitive decline are turning to peptides to enhance focus, memory, and mental clarity. The versatility and effectiveness of peptide bioregulators make them a valuable tool in promoting overall well-being.

As the interest in peptide bioregulators continues to grow, it is essential to recognize their unique position in the health and wellness landscape. Unlike traditional pharmaceuticals that often carry the risk of adverse effects, peptide bioregulators offer a safer alternative with their natural origin and targeted action. Furthermore, their ability to modulate various biological processes makes them suitable for addressing multiple health concerns simultaneously. This holistic approach aligns with the increasing demand for personalized and integrative health solutions.

The historical journey of peptide bioregulators from their initial discovery to their current prominence highlights the transformative potential of these compounds. Early research laid the foundation for understanding their roles in health, while modern advancements have expanded their applications. Today, peptide bioregulators hold promise for enhancing wellness, managing age-related issues, and optimizing performance. By integrating peptide bioregulators into health strategies, individuals can harness the power of these natural compounds to improve their quality of life.

Current Trends and Interest

The renewed interest in peptide bioregulators within health, wellness, and performance enhancement sectors can be attributed to several factors. Firstly, advancements in scientific research have increased our understanding of these naturally occurring compounds. Peptide bioregulators are essentially short chains of amino acids that play crucial roles in maintaining and regulating biological functions. As more studies illuminate their mechanisms and benefits, both consumers and scientists are becoming increasingly intrigued by their potential.

One significant contributor to the growing interest is the shift from traditional pharmaceuticals to natural alternatives. Many individuals are now seeking options that promise fewer side effects and more holistic approaches to health management. The pharmaceutical industry has long been dominated by synthetic drugs, which, while effective, often come with a range of adverse effects and dependency issues. In contrast, peptide bioregulators offer a more natural solution, leveraging the body's inherent biological processes to promote healing and well-being.

This trend towards natural alternatives also aligns with a broader movement in consumer behavior. Health enthusiasts, athletes, and busy professionals alike are turning to supplements and treatments that support overall wellness without compromising their bodies with harsh chemicals. For instance, peptides like collagen are already widely recognized for their benefits to skin health and joint function, further cementing the appeal of bioregulators.

The implications of this trend for future health practices are profound. As more people embrace peptide bioregulators, we may see a paradigm shift in how we approach illness prevention and health optimization. This could lead to a decreased reliance on conventional medicine and an increased focus on proactive, preventative measures. Furthermore, peptides might become integral components of personalized medicine, tailored to meet individual health needs based on genetic and lifestyle factors.

Ongoing research efforts continue to unlock the full potential of peptide bioregulators. Scientists are investigating their applications across various domains, from anti-aging therapies to muscle recovery and cognitive enhancement. For example, thymosin beta-4 is being studied for its regenerative properties in tissue repair, while other peptides are being explored for their neuroprotective effects. These findings not only bolster the credibility of peptide bioregulators but also expand their possible uses in medical and wellness practices.

In the realm of sports and fitness, peptides are garnering attention for their ability to enhance performance, accelerate muscle growth, and improve recovery times. Athletes and fitness aficionados are particularly drawn to these benefits, seeking non-invasive methods to boost their physical capabilities. Growth hormone-releasing peptides (GHRPs), for instance, stimulate the release of growth hormone, which can contribute to increased muscle mass and reduced body fat. Such outcomes are highly desirable in competitive sports and bodybuilding communities.

Moreover, the cognitive benefits of peptide bioregulators are becoming a focal point for many researchers. Busy professionals concerned about cognitive decline are exploring peptides like nootropics to enhance focus, memory, and mental clarity. Nootropic peptides, such as Cerebrolysin, have shown promise in improving cognitive function and protecting against neurodegenerative diseases. These developments highlight the versatility of peptides in addressing diverse health concerns.

While the commercial interest in peptide-based products grows, it is underpinned by rigorous scientific investigation. Researchers are continually conducting clinical trials to verify the efficacy and safety of various peptides. This scientific backing is crucial in establishing trust among consumers and healthcare providers alike. For instance, clinical studies on BPC-157, a peptide known for its healing properties, have demonstrated its potential in treating inflammatory conditions and promoting tissue regeneration.

The integration of peptide bioregulators into mainstream health practices represents a confluence of scientific innovation and consumer demand. With ongoing research and increasing awareness, peptides are poised to redefine the landscape of health and wellness. As our understanding deepens, so too will the applications and benefits of these remarkable compounds.

Looking forward, the future of peptide bioregulators appears promising. Continued advancements in biotechnology and molecular biology will likely yield more potent and specific peptides tailored to address particular health challenges. This will not only enhance the efficacy of treatments but also minimize potential side effects, making peptides an even more attractive option for health-conscious individuals.

Furthermore, collaborations between researchers, healthcare practitioners, and the pharmaceutical industry will be pivotal in advancing the field. Such collaborations can facilitate the translation of laboratory findings into practical applications, ensuring that the benefits of peptides are accessible to a broader audience. Educational initiatives aimed at informing the public and medical community about the advantages and safe use of peptide bioregulators will also play a key role in their widespread adoption.

Role in Longevity and Performance

Peptide bioregulators are increasingly discussed in modern conversations around anti-aging and performance optimization. As the global wellness movement grows, these small proteins are gaining significant traction for their potential benefits. Their ability to influence various biological processes places them at the forefront of current scientific exploration and practical application.

The scientific community has been focusing on peptides because they offer a more natural approach to health enhancement compared to traditional pharmaceuticals. Researchers have found that peptide bioregulators can modulate bodily functions in ways that promote longevity and vitality. For example, peptides like thymosin alpha-1 have shown promise in enhancing immune function, which is crucial for maintaining good health as we age. Similarly, collagen peptides are widely used for improving skin elasticity and reducing wrinkles, making them popular in anti-aging skincare.

Understanding the role of these peptides is essential in the quest for longevity and vitality. By interacting with specific receptors in the body, peptides can influence processes such as hormone regulation, cell repair, and metabolic function. This makes them valuable tools not only for extending lifespan but also for improving the quality of life. For instance, growth hormone-releasing peptides (GHRPs) stimulate the release of growth hormone, aiding muscle growth and recovery, which is particularly beneficial for athletes and fitness enthusiasts.

Providing examples of successful applications in clinical settings further underscores the significance of peptide bioregulators. In medicine, certain peptides are used to treat age-related conditions such as osteoporosis and sarcopenia—conditions characterized by the loss of bone density and muscle mass, respectively. Peptides like calcitonin gene-related peptide (CGRP) have been effective in managing chronic pain conditions, including migraines and cluster headaches.

These clinical successes highlight the therapeutic potential of peptide bioregulators in addressing health issues that commonly arise with aging.

Peptides also show promise in complementing traditional medical treatments. For example, cancer patients undergoing chemotherapy may benefit from the protective effects of peptides like thymosin beta-4, which helps in tissue regeneration and wound healing. Similarly, insulin-like growth factor 1 (IGF-1) can be used alongside conventional diabetes treatments to enhance glucose regulation and improve overall metabolic health. These complementary uses not only enhance the effectiveness of standard treatments but also contribute to better patient outcomes.

The integration of peptide bioregulators into broader health and wellness practices highlights their versatility. From dietary supplements aimed at boosting athletic performance to cosmetic products targeting skin rejuvenation, peptides are becoming integral components of holistic health strategies. Brands are increasingly incorporating peptides into their formulations to meet consumer demand for effective and science-backed solutions. For instance, peptides like BPC-157 are being explored for their potential to expedite muscle recovery and reduce inflammation, appealing to both athletes and individuals with chronic pain conditions.

Moreover, the growing interest in personalized medicine has paved the way for the tailored use of peptide bioregulators based on individual genetic profiles. This personalized approach allows for more precise interventions, maximizing the benefits while minimizing potential side effects. As research progresses, we can expect to see more targeted peptide therapies designed to address specific health needs, thereby revolutionizing the way we manage health and wellness.

Peptide Bioregulators in Therapy

Peptide bioregulators have emerged as a promising avenue in the management of age-related diseases and enhancement of biological functions. These small chains of amino acids play critical roles in health, acting as signaling molecules that regulate various processes within the body. Their therapeutic potential has been explored across a range of health conditions, providing hope for both patients and healthcare providers.

In recent years, there has been a growing interest in the use of peptide bioregulators to combat specific age-related diseases. One noteworthy success is in managing cardiovascular diseases. Peptides like epitalon have shown promise in reducing oxidative stress and improving heart function by activating telomerase, which maintains the length of telomeres—protective caps on chromosomes that shorten with age. This action helps to delay cellular aging and reduce the risk of heart conditions.

Another significant area where peptides have made an impact is neurodegenerative diseases, such as Alzheimer's and Parkinson's. Various neuropeptides have been studied for their neuroprotective properties. For instance, cerebrolysin, a mixture of peptides derived from pig brain proteins, has demonstrated potential in improving cognitive functions and slowing down the progression of Alzheimer's disease. By enhancing neuronal survival and synaptic plasticity, these peptides offer a novel approach to treating conditions that currently have limited therapeutic options.

Peptide bioregulators are also being utilized in endocrine disorders. Thymosin alpha-1, for example, aids in modulating the immune response and has been used in treating autoimmune diseases like multiple sclerosis and rheumatoid arthritis. Its ability to enhance T-cell function makes it a valuable tool in restoring immune balance. Similarly, insulin-like growth factor-1 (IGF-1) plays a crucial role in metabolic regulation and has been beneficial in managing diabetes by improving glucose uptake and reducing insulin resistance.

The journey of peptides from discovery to clinical application has been marked by several scientific milestones. Initial peptide research focused primarily on understanding their basic biological functions. The discovery of insulin in the early 20th century was a groundbreaking event that highlighted the potential of peptides as therapeutic agents. Subsequent decades saw the isolation and synthesis of other significant peptides, such as oxytocin and vasopressin, which further underscored their therapeutic value.

Advancements in peptide synthesis techniques, particularly solid-phase peptide synthesis (SPPS), revolutionized the field by enabling the production of complex peptides with high purity. This technological leap facilitated more rigorous experimentation and the development of peptide-based drugs. Additionally, the advent of recombinant DNA technology allowed for the mass production of peptide hormones, like human growth hormone (HGH), making them more accessible for clinical use.

As our understanding of peptide bioregulators deepens, future trends suggest exciting possibilities for health and wellness. Personalized medicine is one of the most anticipated advancements, where peptide therapies could be tailored to individual genetic profiles and specific health needs. This approach promises greater efficacy and reduced side effects, marking a shift towards more precise and individualized healthcare solutions.

Additionally, regenerative medicine, which aims to repair or replace damaged tissues, stands to benefit significantly from peptide bioregulators. Peptides that promote cell proliferation and differentiation, such as transforming growth factor-beta (TGF-β), could be pivotal in developing treatments for injuries and degenerative diseases. The integration of peptides into stem cell therapy protocols is another area of active research, with the potential to unlock new regenerative capacities.

Despite the progress and potential, the field of peptide bioregulators faces several challenges. One of the primary obstacles is the stability of peptides. Many peptides are susceptible to degradation by enzymes in the body, which limits their bioavailability and effectiveness. Researchers are continually exploring strategies to enhance peptide stability, such as incorporating non-natural amino acids or designing peptide analogs that resist enzymatic breakdown.

Manufacturing and scalability pose additional hurdles. The production of high-quality peptides often requires sophisticated equipment and stringent quality control measures, making it a resource-intensive process. Ensuring consistent batch-to-batch quality is crucial for regulatory approval and market acceptance. Advances in biotechnological methods, however, are gradually addressing these challenges, offering more efficient and cost-effective production solutions.

Safety and regulatory considerations also remain paramount. As peptides interact intricately with biological systems, thorough preclinical and clinical testing is essential to assess their safety profiles. Regulatory bodies, such as the FDA, have established rigorous guidelines for the approval of peptide-based therapies. Navigating these regulatory landscapes can be complex and time-consuming, necessitating a robust framework for clinical trials and documentation.

Public perception and education about peptide bioregulators are equally important. There is a need for increased awareness and understanding among both healthcare professionals and the general public regarding the benefits and limitations of peptide therapies. Clear communication of scientific evidence and realistic expectations can help mitigate misconceptions and foster informed decision-making.

Innovation in Health Supplements

The integration of peptide bioregulators into health supplements and wellness products has seen a notable rise in popularity. This surge is largely due to growing consumer awareness and demand for more effective alternatives to traditional health solutions. Peptide-based supplements are becoming a significant sector of the health industry, driven by promises of enhanced performance, anti-aging benefits, and overall well-being.

Consumers today are highly informed and always on the lookout for innovative and natural ways to improve their health. This shift towards natural and scientifically-backed supplements has opened doors for peptide bioregulators. These short chains of amino acids are known to play crucial roles in regulating various biological functions, making them attractive for those seeking comprehensive wellness solutions. The market growth of these products has been supported by an increasing number of studies highlighting their effectiveness.

One area that shows substantial promise with peptide bioregulators is regenerative medicine. Regenerative medicine aims to replace or regenerate human cells, tissues, or organs to restore normal function. Peptide bioregulators have been found to aid in cellular repair and regeneration, contributing to tissue health and longevity. For example, peptides such as GHK-Cu have shown potential in wound healing and skin regeneration, making them popular in both medical treatments and cosmetic products.

Personalized healthcare is another promising field benefiting from peptide bioregulators. As the concept of customized treatment plans gains traction, peptides offer precise and targeted therapeutic benefits. They can be tailored to meet individual health needs, making healthcare more efficient and personalized. For instance, specific peptides can be formulated to enhance cognitive function in busy professionals, while others may focus on muscle recovery for athletes.

Despite the optimistic outlook, researchers and manufacturers face several challenges in integrating peptide bioregulators into supplements and wellness products. One major challenge is ensuring the stability and bioavailability of peptides when consumed. Peptides can be easily broken down by the digestive system, reducing their effectiveness. To overcome this, advanced delivery systems like encapsulation, transdermal patches, and nasal sprays are being developed to enhance peptide absorption.

Another challenge lies in the regulatory landscape governing the use of peptide bioregulators. Regulatory bodies have stringent requirements for approving new supplements, ensuring they are safe and effective for consumer use. Navigating these regulations can be complex and time-consuming, often requiring significant investment in clinical trials and research. Manufacturers must also ensure consistency in product quality and potency, which can be difficult given the sensitive nature of peptides.

Moreover, there is still a need for more extensive research to fully understand the long-term effects and potential side effects of peptide-based supplements. While preliminary studies show promising results, comprehensive clinical trials are necessary to establish safety profiles and optimal dosages. Researchers are continually exploring different peptide formulations and their impacts on various health conditions to provide more evidence-based recommendations.

In this chapter, we have explored the fundamental nature of peptide bioregulators and their crucial roles in maintaining human health. By delving into their definition and history, we gained insights into how these short chains of amino acids regulate various biological functions. Unlike traditional pharmaceuticals, peptide bioregulators offer a more natural approach to health management, seamlessly integrating with the body's systems to modulate cellular processes without significant side effects. The historical journey from the discovery of insulin to modern advancements has highlighted the transformative potential of peptides in both medical and wellness applications.

Furthermore, current trends underscore the growing interest in peptide bioregulators due to their effectiveness and minimal adverse effects. As scientific research continues to uncover new peptides and their mechanisms, these naturally occurring compounds are being integrated into various health strategies, from enhancing athletic performance to promoting cognitive function and longevity. The versatile nature of peptide bioregulators aligns well with the increasing demand for holistic and personalized health solutions. Overall, the chapter emphasizes the significance of peptides in revolutionizing health practices and improving the quality of life across diverse populations.

CHAPTER 2

The Science Behind Peptide Bioregulators

Peptide bioregulators are small chains of amino acids that play vital roles in the body by acting as messengers between cells. These molecules influence a wide variety of biological processes at the cellular level, contributing to the overall harmony and functionality of our body's systems. By understanding how these peptides work, one can gain valuable insights into their potential benefits for health, performance, and well-being. This chapter delves into the intricate mechanisms through which peptide bioregulators exert their effects within the body.

The chapter thoroughly explains essential biochemical processes involving peptide bioregulators, starting with cell signaling mechanisms. It explores how these peptides interact with specific receptors on cell surfaces, triggering a series of intracellular events that lead to various physiological responses. Next, the chapter discusses gene expression modulation, detailing how peptide bioregulators can upregulate or downregulate certain genes, thereby influencing protein synthesis. Further, it covers the role of peptide bioregulators in protein synthesis facilitation, essential for muscle repair and growth, particularly for athletes. The concept of regulatory feedback loops is also examined, highlighting how these peptides help maintain homeostasis in the body. By the end of this chapter, readers will have a comprehensive understanding of the multifaceted roles of peptide bioregulators in maintaining and enhancing bodily functions.

How Peptide Bioregulators Function

Peptide bioregulators are fascinating molecules that play critical roles in our body's complex biological systems. These small chains of amino acids, often shorter than traditional proteins, act as messengers that transmit vital information between cells to orchestrate a range of physiological responses. Understanding how peptide bioregulators function can enhance our appreciation of their potential in health and performance optimization.

One core mechanism through which peptide bioregulators exert their influence is through cell signaling pathways. These peptides interact with specific receptors on the surfaces of cells, much like a key fitting into a lock. Once a peptide binds to its receptor, it triggers a cascade of intracellular events that ultimately lead to alterations in the cell's behavior. For example, when a peptide bioregulator binds to a cell receptor, it might initiate processes such as muscle contraction, immune response activation, or hormone secretion. This signaling process is crucial for transmitting precise instructions that help maintain the body's operational harmony.

Gene expression modulation is another significant role played by peptide bioregulators. These molecules have the capacity to affect the transcription of particular genes, thereby influencing the production of specific proteins within the body. Gene expression is the process by which information from a gene is used to construct functional products like proteins. When peptide bioregulators modulate this process, they can turn certain genes on or off, leading to increased or decreased protein synthesis. This ability to regulate gene expression allows peptides to impact a wide array of biological functions, including cell growth, metabolism, and repair mechanisms. For instance, some peptide bioregulators may activate genes involved in muscle growth, making them highly beneficial for athletes looking to enhance muscle mass and strength.

In addition to influencing gene expression, peptide bioregulators facilitate protein synthesis directly. Proteins are essential macromolecules required for virtually every function within the human body, from building cellular structures to enabling biochemical reactions. Peptide bioregulators can enhance the efficiency and rate of protein synthesis, ensuring that the body remains equipped with the necessary proteins for diverse physiological activities. For athletes, this translates to improved muscle recovery and growth after intense physical exercise. For individuals focused on anti-aging, efficient protein synthesis helps maintain skin elasticity and repair tissues, contributing to overall wellness and longevity.

Regulatory feedback loops further illustrate the critical role of peptide bioregulators in maintaining homeostasis, which is the body's ability to sustain a stable internal environment despite external changes. Peptide bioregulators participate in various feedback systems that fine-tune and balance biological processes, ensuring they operate within optimal parameters. For example, in the endocrine system, peptide hormones like insulin are involved in feedback loops that control blood glucose levels. When blood sugar rises, insulin is released to facilitate glucose uptake by cells, thereby lowering blood sugar back to normal levels. In scenarios where feedback mechanisms involving peptide bioregulators function efficiently, the result is a balanced state of health and well-being.

Understanding these mechanisms provides valuable insights into how peptide bioregulators can be harnessed for therapeutic purposes. By targeting specific signaling pathways and gene expression profiles, it is possible to design peptide-based interventions that address particular health concerns. For instance, synthetic peptides mimicking natural peptide bioregulators could be developed to treat conditions such as immune deficiencies, metabolic disorders, or even cognitive decline. Additionally, recognizing the role of peptide bioregulators in feedback regulation highlights their potential in crafting personalized medicine approaches aimed at optimizing individual health outcomes.

For health enthusiasts seeking anti-aging solutions, the science behind peptide bioregulators offers promising avenues for enhancing vitality and longevity. The ability of these peptides to modulate gene expression and promote protein synthesis means they can support skin health, muscle maintenance, and tissue repair—key factors in mitigating the effects of aging. Athletes stand to benefit significantly from the performance-enhancing properties of peptide bioregulators. Improved protein synthesis facilitates quicker recovery times, increased muscle mass, and enhanced endurance, all of which contribute to better athletic performance. Busy professionals concerned about cognitive decline may find solace in peptide bioregulators' potential to influence brain function through neuropeptides, thus improving focus, memory, and mental clarity. Lastly, those interested in holistic health approaches can appreciate how peptide bioregulators work synergistically within the body's natural systems, offering a balanced method of achieving wellness without relying on invasive treatments.

Cell Signaling Mechanisms

Peptide bioregulators operate through cell signaling pathways, a critical biochemical process that facilitates communication between cells and orchestrates a wide array of physiological functions. At the heart of these interactions are peptides, short chains of amino acids that bind to specific cell receptors to initiate cellular responses. This binding activity is like fitting a key into a lock—each peptide has a unique structure that allows it to interact specifically with its corresponding receptor on the cell surface.

When a peptide binds to its designated receptor, it triggers a series of intracellular events known as signal transduction. These events often involve the activation of various proteins and secondary messengers within the cell. For instance, the binding can activate enzymes that then convert inactive molecules into active forms, propagating the signal further within the cell. This cascade effect is pivotal in translating the extracellular signal (the peptide binding) into a meaningful intracellular response, ultimately leading to changes in the cell's behavior or function.

Understanding these pathways sheds light on how peptides modulate physiological responses. By knowing which pathways are triggered by specific peptides, researchers can predict how these molecules will influence various biological processes. For example, peptides that bind to receptors on muscle cells might trigger pathways that promote protein synthesis and muscle growth. Conversely, those interacting with immune cells could modulate immune responses, enhancing or dampening the body's defense mechanisms depending on the need.

Receptor activation dynamics also play a crucial role in the precision of peptide actions in targeted tissues. The speed, duration, and intensity of receptor activation determine how effectively a peptide can exert its influence. Some peptides have rapid, short-lived effects, activating their receptors quickly and causing immediate cellular changes. Others may induce prolonged receptor activation, leading to sustained cellular responses. This precision ensures that peptides exert their effects only when and where they are needed, minimizing unintended consequences and optimizing physiological outcomes.

The insights gained from studying cell signaling pathways inspire innovative therapeutic strategies for health optimization. For instance, understanding how specific peptides interact with receptors involved in inflammation has led to the development of anti-inflammatory therapies that target these pathways. Similarly, peptides that influence metabolic pathways are being explored for their potential in managing conditions like obesity and diabetes. By harnessing the power of peptide signaling, scientists and medical professionals can devise treatments that are both precise and effective, offering new avenues for enhancing health and wellness.

One practical application of this knowledge lies in the realm of sports and fitness. Athletes and fitness enthusiasts seek natural methods to improve performance, muscle growth, and recovery times. Peptides that activate receptors involved in muscle repair and regeneration can be used to develop supplements or therapies that enhance muscle recovery post-exercise. This not only aids in faster recovery but also contributes to overall muscle health and performance enhancement.

Busy professionals concerned about cognitive decline can also benefit from peptide research. Certain peptides interact with receptors in the brain to support neuroplasticity and cognitive function. By targeting these pathways, it becomes possible to develop interventions that enhance focus, memory, and mental clarity. Such advancements hold promise for mitigating age-related cognitive decline, helping professionals maintain peak mental performance.

Moreover, individuals interested in holistic health approaches can find value in peptide-based therapies. Alternative medicine often emphasizes the body's natural ability to heal and maintain balance. Peptide bioregulators fit well within this philosophy, as they work by naturally modulating biological processes to restore and maintain homeostasis. For example, peptides that regulate inflammatory pathways can help manage chronic inflammation, a common underlying factor in many health conditions.

Gene Expression Modulation

Peptide bioregulators play a pivotal role in the regulation of gene expression, influencing various biological processes at a molecular level. By altering the transcription of specific genes, these small protein fragments can significantly impact protein synthesis within the body. This modification is crucial for understanding how peptide supplementation can lead to long-term benefits in health and performance.

The process begins with peptides interacting with cellular receptors, which then trigger intracellular signaling pathways leading to changes in gene expression. For instance, when a peptide binds to its receptor on the cell surface, it activates a cascade of events inside the cell that ultimately reaches the nucleus where DNA is stored. Here, the peptide's influence can either upregulate or downregulate the transcription of particular genes. This means that certain genes can be turned on or off, thereby modifying the production of proteins that are essential for various bodily functions.

Understanding how peptides affect gene expression allows us to appreciate their transformative potential, especially in terms of long-term health outcomes. Peptides that promote protein synthesis can support muscle growth, enhance repair mechanisms, and improve overall cellular function. This knowledge empowers individuals to make informed decisions about supplementing with peptides for specific health goals. Whether aiming to build muscle, recover from injury, or improve cognitive function, knowing the underlying mechanisms can guide more effective and personalized approaches to wellness.

The implications of this process are particularly significant in the context of anti-aging and recovery. As we age, the efficiency of our body's cellular functions declines, partly due to a decrease in the production of key proteins. Peptide bioregulators can help counteract these effects by promoting the transcription of genes involved in protein synthesis, thus supporting the maintenance of tissue integrity and function. For example, some peptides have been shown to stimulate the production of collagen, a vital protein for skin elasticity and joint health. By enhancing collagen synthesis, these peptides can help reduce signs of aging and maintain mobility.

Moreover, the interplay between peptides and gene expression offers valuable insights into recovery processes. Following intense physical activity or injury, the body's ability to repair damaged tissues is paramount. Peptides that influence gene expression related to muscle repair and inflammation can accelerate recovery times and reduce soreness. Athletes and fitness enthusiasts, therefore, may find peptide supplementation an effective strategy for improving post-exercise recovery and overall performance. The enhancement of recovery processes not only aids in quicker return to training but also minimizes the risk of overtraining and injury.

Delving deeper into the science reveals that modifying gene expression through peptides can extend beyond physical performance to broader health improvements. For example, peptides that modulate the expression of genes involved in metabolic processes can aid in weight management and metabolic health. By influencing genes that regulate insulin sensitivity and fat metabolism, peptides can help optimize energy utilization and storage, contributing to better overall health outcomes.

Furthermore, peptides with neuroprotective properties highlight the importance of gene expression modulation in cognitive health. Certain peptides can influence the transcription of genes involved in neural growth and synaptic plasticity, which are critical for maintaining cognitive function and preventing decline. These peptides can thus potentially enhance focus, memory, and mental clarity, making them attractive to busy professionals seeking cognitive enhancement.

Given the broad implications of peptide-induced gene expression modifications, it is essential to recognize the diverse range of health and performance benefits they offer. From supporting muscle growth and recovery to promoting anti-aging and cognitive health, peptides provide a multifaceted approach to wellness that leverages fundamental biological processes. Empowering readers with this knowledge enables them to make informed decisions about integrating peptides into their health regimens for optimal results.

Different Types of Peptide Bioregulators

Peptide bioregulators play a crucial role in maintaining and enhancing the various bodily functions that contribute to overall health and well-being. To understand their full potential, it's essential to categorize and describe the different types of peptide bioregulators and highlight their distinct functions.

Hormonal peptides are one significant category. These peptides either mimic or modulate hormone activities in the body, impacting endocrine health and metabolic regulation. Hormonal peptides offer therapeutic potential for conditions such as diabetes by influencing insulin levels, thereby helping regulate blood sugar. Additionally, they assist in managing thyroid function and can be utilized in hormone replacement therapies, presenting promising avenues for treating hormonal imbalances. For fitness enthusiasts, these peptides support muscle growth and energy metabolism, making them valuable for performance enhancement.

Neuropeptides, another vital category, have a profound influence on brain function and emotional responses. These peptides serve as neurotransmitters and neuromodulators, affecting various aspects of mood, cognition, and behavior. For example, the neuropeptide oxytocin is often referred to as the "love hormone" due to its role in social bonding and stress relief. Similarly, endorphins are neuropeptides that act as natural painkillers and mood enhancers, contributing to feelings of euphoria commonly experienced during exercise, also known as the "runner's high." The therapeutic potential of neuropeptides extends to mental health, offering possibilities for treatments of disorders like depression, anxiety, and PTSD by targeting specific neural pathways to improve emotional well-being.

Antimicrobial peptides form a crucial part of the body's innate immune defense system. These peptides possess broad-spectrum activity against bacteria, viruses, fungi, and even some cancers. They function by disrupting the membranes of harmful microorganisms, effectively neutralizing pathogens before they can cause infection. Antimicrobial peptides are being explored as alternatives to traditional antibiotics, offering hope in the battle against antibiotic-resistant superbugs. Their immune-boosting properties make them beneficial not only for general health but also for individuals with weakened immune systems, such as those undergoing chemotherapy or suffering from chronic illnesses.

Growth factors, the final category discussed here, play an instrumental role in stimulating cell growth and regeneration. These peptides signal cells to proliferate, differentiate, and repair tissues, which is critical for healing wounds and recovering from injuries. Growth factors like EGF (epidermal growth factor) and IGF (insulin-like growth factor) are widely studied for their applications in regenerative medicine and anti-aging treatments. Athletes particularly benefit from growth factors as they aid in muscle repair and recovery, reducing downtime and enhancing performance. In cosmetic medicine, these peptides are used in skin rejuvenation therapies, promoting collagen production and reducing the signs of aging.

Protein Synthesis Facilitation and Homeostasis

Peptide bioregulators are small proteins that play a critical role in regulating numerous biological processes in the body. One of their primary functions is to enhance protein synthesis, which is vital for muscle repair and various cellular activities. When the body undergoes physical stress, such as exercise or injury, muscles experience micro-tears that need to be repaired. Peptide bioregulators stimulate the creation of new proteins, facilitating the repair and growth of muscle tissues. This process is particularly important for athletes and fitness enthusiasts who rely on efficient muscle recovery to improve performance and stamina.

The enhanced protein synthesis attributed to peptide bioregulators also contributes to broader bodily functions beyond just muscle repair. Proteins serve as building blocks for cells, enzymes, hormones, and other essential compounds in the body. By boosting protein synthesis, peptides support these critical functions, ensuring that the body's biological systems operate optimally. This aspect of peptides makes them valuable not only for those focused on physical health but also for individuals seeking overall wellness and longevity.

Understanding how peptide bioregulators facilitate muscle repair and growth is crucial for anyone involved in athletic or fitness activities. When muscles endure intense workouts, they require adequate nutrients and biochemical support to recover effectively. Peptide bioregulators provide this support by signaling the body to produce necessary proteins more efficiently. This mechanism helps reduce recovery times and enhances muscle strength, allowing athletes to train harder and achieve better results. Additionally, a well-regulated protein synthesis process helps prevent injuries, making it a cornerstone of any comprehensive fitness regimen.

A key factor in maintaining optimal health is understanding the feedback mechanisms that regulate biological processes. Feedback loops are systems within the body that monitor and adjust physiological functions to maintain homeostasis or internal balance. Peptide bioregulators play a significant role in these feedback mechanisms. For instance, when protein levels in the body are low, peptide bioregulators can signal the need for increased protein synthesis. Conversely, when protein levels are sufficient, these peptides help downregulate production to avoid excess. This regulation ensures that the body remains in a balanced state, preventing conditions caused by either deficiency or surplus of essential proteins.

The concept of feedback mechanisms highlights the importance of balance in health interventions. Whether through diet, exercise, or supplementation, it is essential to strive for equilibrium rather than extremes. Overloading the body with external supplements without understanding its inherent feedback systems can disrupt natural balance, leading to adverse effects. Therefore, education about how peptides work within these feedback loops can inform smarter health decisions and interventions.

Homeostasis is the body's ability to maintain a stable internal environment despite external changes. Peptide bioregulators contribute significantly to this stability by influencing various physiological processes. For example, they assist in regulating blood pressure, glucose levels, and immune responses—all crucial elements of homeostasis. By modulating these functions, peptides help keep the body's internal environment consistent, promoting overall health and well-being.

Furthermore, maintaining biological stability has far-reaching implications for long-term health. Conditions like chronic inflammation, hormonal imbalances, and metabolic disorders often result from disruptions in homeostasis. Peptide bioregulators, by supporting stable and balanced biological processes, can help mitigate these issues. Their role in sustaining homeostasis underscores their potential in preventive healthcare, where the focus is on maintaining health rather than merely treating diseases.

For busy professionals concerned with cognitive decline, peptides' role in maintaining homeostasis is particularly relevant. Cognitive functions such as memory, focus, and mental clarity are heavily dependent on a stable internal environment. Disruption in homeostasis due to stress, poor diet, or lack of sleep can impair cognitive abilities. By supporting the body's regulatory systems, peptide bioregulators contribute to sustained mental performance, making them an attractive option for individuals aiming to enhance cognitive health naturally.

Holistic health approaches often emphasize the interconnectedness of different bodily systems. Peptide bioregulators align well with this philosophy, as they do not target a single function but rather influence multiple aspects of biological stability. By enhancing protein synthesis and participating in feedback mechanisms, peptides support a broad spectrum of bodily functions. This multifaceted approach makes them a valuable component of holistic wellness strategies, where the goal is to promote overall health rather than isolated benefits.

Given the diverse roles of peptide bioregulators, it is evident that they offer significant benefits for various groups of people. From athletes seeking improved performance to professionals aiming for better cognitive function, the ability of peptides to boost protein synthesis and maintain homeostasis makes them a versatile tool in health optimization. Educating oneself about how these small proteins work can empower individuals to make informed choices about their health interventions, aligning with both scientific evidence and personal wellness goals.

This chapter has detailed the biochemical roles and mechanisms of peptide bioregulators in the body, illustrating how these small molecules function at the cellular level to regulate various biological processes. By interacting with cell receptors and influencing gene expression, peptides play a crucial part in signaling pathways that control muscle contraction, immune responses, hormone secretion, and more. This understanding opens the door to using peptide-based interventions for health optimization, from enhancing athletic performance and recovery to supporting anti-aging and cognitive health.

Moreover, the chapter highlighted the importance of peptide bioregulators in maintaining homeostasis and facilitating protein synthesis, which are vital for overall wellness. Whether it's restoring balance through regulatory feedback loops or promoting tissue repair and growth, peptides have significant therapeutic potential. For athletes, they offer improved muscle recovery and growth; for those focused on anti-aging, they support skin elasticity and tissue repair. Busy professionals can benefit from their effects on brain function, while individuals interested in holistic health can appreciate their natural synergy within the body's systems. Understanding these mechanisms allows for informed decisions about incorporating peptides into personalized health strategies.

CHAPTER 3

Anti-Aging with Peptide Bioregulators

Reducing the signs of aging with peptide bioregulators centers on understanding how these molecules can enhance skin elasticity and overall vitality. Peptide bioregulators, which can be either naturally occurring or synthetic, play a pivotal role in regulating various biological processes that directly impact skin health. By interacting with specific cell receptors, these peptides stimulate the production of essential proteins such as collagen. This process is fundamental for maintaining skin firmness and elasticity, crucial elements for youthful-looking skin.

In this chapter, we will explore the different ways peptide bioregulators contribute to improved skin health and vitality. We will delve into how they boost collagen production and support skin hydration, both vital for reducing fine lines and wrinkles. Additionally, the chapter will cover the mechanisms through which peptide bioregulators enhance skin repair processes, ensuring quicker recovery from environmental damage. Lastly, we will examine their antioxidant properties that help mitigate oxidative stress, further supporting long-term skin health and resilience.

Improving Skin Elasticity

Understanding how peptide bioregulators can promote skin health and elasticity is crucial to grasping their role in anti-aging. These molecules are naturally occurring or synthetic peptides that regulate various biological processes, including skin function. By interacting with specific cell receptors, peptide bioregulators can stimulate the production of essential proteins such as collagen, which is vital for maintaining skin firmness and elasticity.

Collagen synthesis is a foundational aspect of healthy, youthful skin. Collagen is a protein that provides structure and strength to the skin. As we age, collagen production decreases, leading to the formation of wrinkles and sagging skin. Peptide bioregulators have been shown to enhance collagen production by activating fibroblasts, the cells responsible for synthesizing collagen. This activation leads to an increase in collagen levels within the skin, helping to restore its firmness and elasticity. When collagen levels are bolstered, the skin's underlying structure becomes stronger and more resilient, effectively reducing the appearance of fine lines and wrinkles.

Enhanced collagen levels lead to smoother skin texture. With increased collagen production, the skin becomes plumper, filling in fine lines and reducing the depth of wrinkles. This results in a smoother, more even skin surface that reflects light better, giving the complexion a more youthful glow. The visible reduction in wrinkles not only enhances aesthetic appeal but also boosts confidence. By regularly incorporating peptide bioregulators into skincare routines, individuals can experience long-term improvements in skin texture and overall appearance.

Hydration is another critical factor in maintaining healthy, youthful skin. Peptide bioregulators play a significant role in promoting skin hydration. Properly hydrated skin appears fuller and more supple, which helps minimize the appearance of fine lines and prevent new ones from forming. These bioregulators work by enhancing the skin's natural ability to retain moisture. They support the function of glycosaminoglycans (GAGs) such as hyaluronic acid, which can hold vast amounts of water. By boosting GAG function, peptide bioregulators ensure that the skin remains adequately hydrated, preserving its plumpness and resilience.

Moreover, hydrated skin is less prone to irritation and damage. Environmental factors like pollution, UV radiation, and extreme weather can dehydrate the skin, making it brittle and more susceptible to injury. Peptide bioregulators help maintain optimal hydration levels, strengthening the skin's barrier function and improving its ability to repair and protect itself. Consequently, well-hydrated skin is better equipped to recover from environmental stressors, maintaining its youthful appearance longer.

Skin repair mechanisms are another area where peptide bioregulators shine. These molecules can accelerate the skin's natural repair processes, aiding quicker recovery from environmental damage. Skin frequently encounters harmful elements such as UV rays, pollutants, and harsh weather conditions, all of which can cause oxidative stress and cellular damage. Peptide bioregulators enhance the activity of enzymes and growth factors involved in skin repair and regeneration, speeding up the healing process.

For example, certain peptide bioregulators can boost the production of elastin, another structural protein that, along with collagen, provides skin with elasticity and resilience. Increased elastin levels help the skin snap back to its original shape after being stretched or stressed. Additionally, these bioregulators can aid in the synthesis of extracellular matrix components, which form the scaffolding that supports skin cells. A robust extracellular matrix is essential for maintaining skin integrity and promoting efficient cell turnover, ensuring that damaged cells are replaced by healthy, new ones.

Furthermore, peptide bioregulators possess antioxidant properties that neutralize free radicals, reducing oxidative stress and preventing further cellular damage. This protective effect is crucial for maintaining skin health, as prolonged oxidative stress can accelerate the aging process and lead to various skin issues, including hyperpigmentation and loss of elasticity. By mitigating oxidative damage, peptide bioregulators not only support skin repair but also contribute to long-term skin health.

Boosting Energy Levels

Peptide bioregulators have emerged as a groundbreaking solution in the realm of anti-aging, primarily due to their ability to enhance physical energy and overall well-being. At the cellular level, these molecules boost energy production, which plays a crucial role in combating fatigue commonly associated with aging. As individuals age, their energy levels often decline due to diminished mitochondrial function—the powerhouse of cells. Peptide bioregulators work by stimulating mitochondrial activity, leading to more efficient energy production. This efficiency translates into enhanced stamina and reduced feelings of tiredness, making daily activities less strenuous.

The benefits of peptide bioregulators extend beyond merely addressing fatigue. Higher energy levels significantly impact daily performance and overall quality of life. When energy levels are optimized, individuals can engage more effectively in both professional and personal tasks. Simple activities such as walking, climbing stairs, or even household chores become easier to manage. For athletes and fitness enthusiasts, this means being able to train harder and recover faster. The ripple effect of improved energy production leads to better endurance, allowing for longer and more intense exercise sessions, which in turn supports muscle growth and cardiovascular health.

Moreover, increased vitality from peptide bioregulators supports an active lifestyle, essential for longevity. Physical activity is a cornerstone of healthy aging; it keeps muscles toned, joints flexible, and maintains healthy body weight. An active lifestyle also contributes to reducing the risk of chronic diseases such as diabetes, hypertension, and osteoporosis. With higher energy levels, older adults can maintain regular exercise routines, partake in recreational sports, and enjoy outdoor activities, all of which contribute to a prolonged life expectancy and healthier aging process.

In addition to enhancing physical capabilities, feeling more energetic encourages social engagement, which is vital for mental health. Social interactions play a crucial role in maintaining cognitive function and emotional well-being, especially in older adults. Regular social activities can help stave off depression, anxiety, and loneliness, common issues that many face as they age. By boosting energy levels, peptide bioregulators enable individuals to participate more actively in social gatherings, volunteer work, or community events. Staying socially active helps build meaningful relationships and provides a sense of purpose, which is integral to a fulfilling life.

Furthermore, the increased energy facilitated by peptide bioregulators creates a positive feedback loop. More energy allows for increased activity levels, which in turn stimulates further energy production within the body. This cycle helps sustain high energy levels over time, creating continuous improvements in physical and mental health. Individuals who experience these benefits are more likely to adopt healthier lifestyles, including balanced diets, regular physical exercise, and engaging hobbies.

The implications for busy professionals and those concerned about cognitive decline are equally significant. Higher physical energy not only enables professionals to handle demanding workloads but also improves focus and productivity. An energetic individual is better equipped to manage stress, meet deadlines, and make critical decisions efficiently. For those battling the cognitive effects of aging, maintaining high energy levels can support better memory retention, quicker problem-solving skills, and greater mental clarity.

Supporting Cognitive Function

Peptide bioregulators have garnered significant attention within the health and wellness community for their potential benefits, not just for physical vitality but also for brain health and cognitive function. Research indicates that certain peptide bioregulators may have a profound impact on mental clarity and decision-making capabilities, which are essential as one ages.

To understand how peptide bioregulators influence brain health, it's important to start with their basic function. These molecules act as signaling agents within the body, typically interacting with DNA to promote the expression of specific proteins. This activity can target various tissues, including those in the brain. Emerging studies suggest that some peptide bioregulators can cross the blood-brain barrier—a critical feature for any compound aiming to affect brain health directly.

One of the notable ways peptide bioregulators contribute to enhanced cognitive function is by supporting neurogenesis, the process through which new neurons are formed in the brain. Neurogenesis is crucial for learning and memory. By stimulating the production of new neurons, peptide bioregulators may help sustain and even improve these cognitive faculties. For instance, peptides such as Epithalon have been shown to upregulate the expression of brain-derived neurotrophic factor (BDNF), a protein closely associated with neurogenesis and synaptic plasticity.

Enhanced cognitive function translates into better decision-making and mental clarity. In practical terms, individuals who benefit from improved brain health find themselves more adept at solving problems, making decisions, and processing information efficiently. Mental clarity ensures that tasks requiring focus and concentration can be performed effectively, which is crucial for professionals juggling multiple responsibilities. For athletes and fitness aficionados, quick decision-making can translate into better performance and optimized training regimens.

A sharper mind does more than just enhance daily productivity; it significantly contributes to overall vitality and engagement with life. When mental faculties are sharp, people generally feel more energetic and motivated to participate in social activities and pursue interests. This engagement fosters an enriching life experience, promoting emotional well-being alongside cognitive health. A well-stimulated mind also encourages lifelong learning, a habit strongly linked to longevity and quality of life.

Maintaining cognitive health is especially crucial as one ages. The risk of cognitive decline increases with age, leading to conditions such as mild cognitive impairment (MCI) and dementia. By potentially staving off these declines, peptide bioregulators play a key role in ensuring a high quality of life well into one's senior years. For health enthusiasts interested in anti-aging solutions, this could mean more years of active, fulfilling living without the burden of significant cognitive deterioration.

Another vital aspect to consider is the holistic approach to health that peptide bioregulators support. Cognitive health doesn't exist in isolation; it is intimately connected with physical and emotional well-being. Enhanced brain health can lead to better sleep patterns, reduced stress levels, and improved physical health outcomes. Busy professionals may find that maintaining cognitive health enables them to manage stress and avoid burnout more effectively. Athletes may experience quicker recovery times and improved coordination, which are direct benefits of a well-functioning brain.

Moreover, the ripple effects of strong cognitive health are far-reaching. A mind that operates at peak performance tends to make healthier lifestyle choices, whether that involves diet, exercise, or social interactions. This domino effect leads to a more balanced life, providing a sturdy foundation for both physical and emotional health. Individuals who take proactive steps to maintain cognitive health often report higher satisfaction levels in various facets of life, reinforcing the idea that a healthy mind is indeed the cornerstone of a healthy life.

While there are numerous supplements and interventions available for enhancing cognitive function, the appeal of peptide bioregulators lies in their natural origin and targeted action. Unlike pharmaceutical drugs that might carry significant side effects, peptide bioregulators typically exhibit fewer adverse reactions due to their compatibility with the body's natural processes. This makes them an attractive option for those keen on a more natural approach to maintaining brain health.

It's also pertinent to understand that the benefits of peptide bioregulators extend beyond immediate cognitive enhancements. Long-term use may contribute to sustained mental acuity, providing a buffer against age-related cognitive decline. Continuous improvement and maintenance of cognitive functions ensure that individuals remain mentally agile, capable of adapting to new challenges, and enjoying a high quality of life.

Enhancing Metabolic Processes

Peptide bioregulators are emerging as pivotal components in optimizing metabolism for healthy aging. These small molecules play a significant role in balancing energy expenditure and intake, essential aspects of maintaining a robust metabolic system. For individuals aiming to age gracefully while retaining physical vitality and cognitive sharpness, understanding how peptide bioregulators impact these processes is crucial.

Healthy metabolism is the backbone of overall wellness, influencing everything from weight management to energy levels. Peptide bioregulators contribute by fine-tuning the body's energy expenditure and intake balance. This regulation ensures that the calories consumed are effectively utilized, reducing the accumulation of excess fat, which is commonly associated with aging. As the body ages, metabolic rates naturally decline, leading to potential weight gain and related health complications such as diabetes and cardiovascular diseases. By assisting in balancing these energy dynamics, peptide bioregulators help mitigate these risks.

One of the primary benefits of optimal metabolism is the reduction in age-related weight gain. Maintaining a healthy weight as one ages is a common challenge due to slower metabolic rates. However, peptide bioregulators can help counteract this slowdown. They enhance the body's ability to burn calories efficiently, ensuring that energy produced from food intake is properly expended. This not only helps in avoiding unwanted weight gain but also prevents the onset of various metabolic disorders that become more prevalent with age.

Efficient nutrient utilization is another critical factor influenced by peptide bioregulators. As people age, their bodies often become less efficient at absorbing and utilizing nutrients, leading to deficiencies that can affect overall vitality and health. Peptide bioregulators improve the body's capacity to extract and use vital nutrients from food. This enhanced nutrient absorption supports sustained physical activity, an essential component of healthy aging. Incorporating regular exercise into one's lifestyle is significantly easier when the body is primed to make the most of the nutrients it receives, thereby boosting energy levels and endurance.

Moreover, a well-functioning metabolism is fundamental to maintaining a healthy weight, contributing directly to overall well-being and longevity. The connection between metabolism and weight is intricate; a sluggish metabolic rate often results in weight gain, while a hyperactive metabolism can lead to unhealthy weight loss. Peptide bioregulators strike a balance, ensuring that the metabolic rate remains within optimal ranges relevant to individual needs. This balanced metabolism supports other bodily functions, including hormone regulation and immune responses, creating a ripple effect of health benefits.

It is worth noting the indirect benefits of a well-regulated metabolism facilitated by peptide bioregulators. With improved metabolic efficiency, the body experiences increased energy levels, translating into better physical performance and stamina. For athletes and fitness enthusiasts, this means enhanced muscle growth, quicker recovery times, and more effective training sessions. For busy professionals or those keen on maintaining cognitive function, the energy boost provided by an optimized metabolism can enhance focus, memory, and mental clarity, crucial elements for productivity and overall mental agility.

Furthermore, an optimized metabolism impacts hormonal balance, a key factor in aging and general health. Hormones influence numerous body functions, from mood to sleep patterns and even skin health. By stabilizing metabolic processes, peptide bioregulators indirectly support hormonal health, reducing the chances of hormonal imbalances that could lead to various health issues. Improved hormone regulation also enhances the body's natural repair mechanisms, promoting healthier aging by keeping skin resilient and youthful and supporting the maintenance of lean muscle mass.

Incorporating peptide bioregulators into daily health routines offers a proactive approach to managing aging-related metabolic changes. These molecules can be especially beneficial when combined with other healthy lifestyle practices such as balanced diets and regular exercise. Together, they create a synergistic effect that maximizes the body's natural capabilities, fostering an environment where aging does not equate to a decline in quality of life but rather a period of sustained vitality and enhanced well-being.

For those interested in holistic health approaches, peptide bioregulators present a compelling, natural method to support metabolism and, consequently, healthy aging. Unlike synthetic supplements or invasive procedures, these bioregulators work harmoniously with the body's existing systems. Their use aligns with the principles of alternative medicine, emphasizing prevention and natural healing over symptom treatment.

Stress Management Assistance

Peptide bioregulators are gaining reputation as a powerful tool in managing stress and promoting overall wellness. These tiny molecules, found naturally in the body and also available in supplement form, influence various bodily processes, including how the body handles stress. By regulating stress more effectively, peptide bioregulators can mitigate the impacts of chronic stress, leading to significant health benefits.

Chronic stress poses multiple threats to physical and mental health. It can trigger inflammation, disrupt sleep, weaken the immune system, and even accelerate aging processes. Stress management is essential to maintain optimal health, and peptide bioregulators play a crucial role in this regard. These molecules help regulate the body's stress response through mechanisms like balancing hormones and improving cellular communication. This helps the body transition from a stressed state to a relaxed one more smoothly, thereby mitigating the adverse effects of prolonged stress.

Lowering stress levels has a domino effect on overall well-being. When your body handles stress more efficiently, you experience improved mental clarity, better mood, and increased energy levels. This is especially important for individuals with high-stress lifestyles such as busy professionals or athletes who often face physical and mental strain. Reducing stress supports a balanced state of mind, allowing for clearer thinking and better decision-making, which translates to more productivity and enhanced focus.

Moreover, physical health also sees substantial benefits from lower stress levels. Studies have shown that effective stress management leads to better cardiovascular health by maintaining healthy blood pressure levels and reducing the risk of heart diseases. The immune system functions more robustly, making the body less susceptible to illnesses and infections. Essentially, when the body is not constantly fighting stress, it can divert its resources to healing and maintaining other vital functions.

Reduced stress levels also enhance recovery and resilience against age-related decline. For athletes and fitness enthusiasts, quicker recovery times and enhanced resilience mean more effective training sessions and improved performance. Stress is known to delay muscle recovery and increase the risk of injuries due to heightened cortisol levels. By managing stress effectively, peptide bioregulators help reduce cortisol spikes, fostering an environment where muscles can repair and grow more efficiently.

The impact on mental health cannot be understated either. Lowered stress levels contribute to a more stable emotional state, which is vital for long-term mental wellness. Chronic stress is linked to anxiety, depression, and cognitive decline. By mitigating these stress effects, peptide bioregulators support mental health, which is crucial for anyone looking to maintain their cognitive abilities as they age. Busy professionals, in particular, benefit from enhanced focus and memory retention, attributes that are directly linked to effective stress management.

Effective stress management fosters a vibrant and healthier lifestyle. When stress is under control, you feel more energetic and motivated to engage in activities that contribute to overall wellness. Whether it is partaking in regular exercise, engaging in social activities, or pursuing hobbies, managing stress allows you to live a balanced and fulfilling life. Social interactions and hobbies are particularly beneficial as they provide emotional satisfaction and mental stimulation, both of which are essential for a healthy, long life.

In summary, peptide bioregulators offer a promising solution for stress management, yielding multiple health benefits. They help the body handle stress more efficiently, which mitigates the adverse effects of chronic stress on physical and mental health. Reduced stress levels lead to better overall wellness, as evidenced by improved mental clarity, enhanced physical health, quicker recovery rates, and a more stable emotional state. By integrating peptide bioregulators into stress management strategies, individuals can promote a vibrant and healthier lifestyle, enhancing their quality of life and longevity.

This chapter has delved into the significant role of peptide bioregulators in mitigating signs of aging, particularly through their ability to enhance skin elasticity and overall vitality. By boosting collagen production and supporting optimal hydration, these molecules strengthen the skin's structure, making it more resilient and reducing the appearance of fine lines and wrinkles. Additionally, the antioxidant properties of peptide bioregulators help protect against oxidative stress, further contributing to long-term skin health.

Moreover, peptide bioregulators extend their benefits beyond skin health by enhancing energy levels and promoting quicker recovery from environmental damage. Their positive impact on mitochondrial function translates to improved stamina and reduced fatigue, enabling a more active lifestyle. As a result, individuals can maintain physical activities with greater ease, leading to long-lasting improvements in both appearance and well-being. Integrating peptide bioregulators into daily routines presents a promising approach for those seeking natural, effective solutions for aging gracefully.

CHAPTER 4

Performance Enhancement for Athletes

E nhancing athletic performance is a goal shared by many athletes and fitness enthusiasts. One of the natural methods gaining attention in this field is the use of peptide bioregulators. These compounds are known for their ability to support muscle growth and improve endurance, thus providing a holistic approach to boosting performance. By understanding how these bioregulators can be integrated into training regimens, athletes can achieve significant improvements in their strength, stamina, and overall athletic ability.

In this chapter, readers will explore the various benefits of peptide bioregulators, specifically focusing on two main areas: muscle growth and endurance improvement. The discussion will cover how these peptides enhance protein synthesis, improve nitrogen retention, expedite recovery from intense workouts, and inhibit muscle breakdown. Additionally, the chapter will delve into how peptide bioregulators can increase aerobic capacity, optimize energy metabolism, and reduce lactic acid build-up, thereby enhancing endurance. Through this exploration, athletes and fitness aficionados will gain valuable insights into how to naturally and effectively boost their performance using peptide bioregulators.

Muscle Growth

Peptide bioregulators have emerged as a powerful tool for athletes looking to boost their performance naturally. One of the primary ways these substances enhance athletic output is by facilitating muscle growth.

Increased Protein Synthesis

A key benefit of peptide bioregulators is their ability to enhance protein synthesis within the body. Proteins serve as the building blocks of muscles, and the rate at which protein is synthesized directly impacts muscle growth. When an athlete engages in strenuous training, muscle fibers experience micro-tears. To repair these tears and build stronger muscles, the body must synthesize new proteins. Peptide bioregulators optimize this process, ensuring that the body can generate proteins more efficiently. This accelerated protein synthesis means that athletes can achieve greater muscle gain in a shorter period.

Protein synthesis is not just about muscle gain; it's also critical for recovery. Enhanced muscle repair processes are crucial for athletes who subject their bodies to strain. When the muscle repair mechanism is optimized, athletes can train harder and longer without the same level of fatigue. Athletes can leverage this response to maximize their training efforts, leading to better outcomes in terms of strength and endurance.

Improved Nitrogen Retention

Another significant advantage of peptide bioregulators is their ability to improve nitrogen retention. Nitrogen is a fundamental component of amino acids, which in turn are the building blocks of proteins. For muscles to grow and repair effectively, maintaining a positive nitrogen balance is crucial. When the body retains more nitrogen, it signals an anabolic state—a condition where muscle building outpaces muscle breakdown.

Peptide bioregulators support this anabolic environment by enhancing the body's ability to hold onto nitrogen. This improved nitrogen retention contributes to muscle anabolism, making it easier for athletes to maintain and build muscle mass. Maintaining a positive nitrogen balance is especially beneficial during periods of intense training or dieting, where muscle preservation is essential. By helping the body retain nitrogen, peptide bioregulators ensure that athletes' muscles remain in an optimal state for growth and recovery.

Enhanced Recovery from Routines

Recovery is another area where peptide bioregulators offer immense benefits. Intense workouts put a significant amount of stress on the muscles, often leading to soreness and fatigue. Traditional methods of recovery, such as rest and nutrition, are effective but can be time-consuming. Peptide bioregulators expedite the recovery process, enabling athletes to return to their training regimens much faster.

These bioregulators work by speeding up the repair of damaged muscle tissue and reducing inflammation. Faster recovery times mean that athletes can engage in more frequent and intense training sessions without suffering from prolonged downtime due to muscle soreness. This capacity to recover rapidly is invaluable for athletes who need to maintain peak performance levels consistently. Additionally, quicker recovery reduces the risk of overtraining, which can lead to injuries and long-term damage.

Inhibition of Muscle Breakdown

Intense workouts and physical activities can lead to muscle catabolism, wherein muscle tissue breaks down faster than it can be repaired. This is particularly detrimental for athletes who rely on muscle strength and endurance. Peptide bioregulators come into play by inhibiting muscle breakdown during high-intensity workouts. Some peptide bioregulators have been shown to possess anti-catabolic properties, meaning they prevent the breakdown of muscle tissue.

By protecting muscles from excessive breakdown, these bioregulators allow athletes to preserve their hard-earned muscle mass even during strenuous exercise. This protection ensures that the gains made during training are not lost due to catabolism. The inhibition of muscle breakdown is crucial for long-term muscle health and performance. It allows athletes to sustain their muscle mass and strength over extended periods, contributing to consistent performance improvements.

The synergistic effects of increased protein synthesis, improved nitrogen retention, expedited recovery, and inhibition of muscle breakdown combine to make peptide bioregulators a potent aid in muscle growth. These mechanisms work together to create a conducive environment for muscle development and maintenance, thereby significantly enhancing athletic performance.

Through more efficient protein synthesis, athletes can see accelerated muscle growth and improved overall recovery. Enhanced nitrogen retention ensures that the body remains in an anabolic state, ideal for muscle building. Faster recovery times mean that athletes can stick to their training schedules without the delays commonly caused by muscle soreness and fatigue. Finally, the inhibition of muscle breakdown preserves the muscle mass that athletes work so hard to build.

Endurance Improvement

Athletic performance can be significantly enhanced through the use of peptide bioregulators, particularly in terms of improving endurance. Endurance is a crucial aspect of athletic prowess, allowing athletes to sustain prolonged physical activity with reduced fatigue. The potential for peptide bioregulators to improve endurance is based on several mechanisms.

Firstly, increased aerobic capacity is one of the primary benefits of peptide bioregulators. Aerobic capacity refers to the body's ability to take in, transport, and utilize oxygen during exercise. Certain peptides stimulate the production of red blood cells, which are responsible for carrying oxygen throughout the body. With more red blood cells, the body can transport oxygen more efficiently to muscles and organs, thereby enhancing overall aerobic performance. This improvement in oxygen delivery not only boosts endurance but also facilitates better overall function of the cardiovascular system.

Beyond improving oxygen delivery, these peptides enhance oxygen utilization within muscle tissues. During prolonged activities like running or cycling, efficient oxygen usage is critical for maintaining energy levels and delaying the onset of fatigue. Peptides work at a cellular level, optimizing the mitochondria's function, which are the powerhouses of cells. Enhanced mitochondrial function means that muscles can produce energy more efficiently, further supporting sustained physical exertion.

Another significant benefit of peptide bioregulators is their role in enhancing recovery from fatigue. Prolonged physical exertion inevitably leads to fatigue, which can hamper performance and prolong recovery times. Peptide bioregulators help mitigate this by aiding the body's recovery processes. They reduce inflammation and promote repair mechanisms within muscle tissues. For instance, some peptides increase the production of growth factors, which are crucial for tissue repair and regeneration. By accelerating the recovery process, athletes can train harder and more frequently without experiencing debilitating fatigue.

Improved energy metabolism is also a notable advantage offered by peptide bioregulators. Energy metabolism involves the process by which the body converts food into usable energy, particularly during exercise. Efficient energy metabolism is essential for sustaining prolonged physical efforts. Peptide bioregulators optimize this process by enhancing the breakdown of stored glycogen and fats into glucose, which is then used as fuel by the muscles. This optimization ensures that athletes have a steady supply of energy throughout their workouts, enabling them to perform at their best for longer periods.

Moreover, peptide bioregulators play a crucial role in reducing lactic acid build-up. Lactic acid is a byproduct of anaerobic metabolism, which occurs when the body produces energy without enough oxygen. High levels of lactic acid can lead to muscle soreness and fatigue, limiting an athlete's performance. Certain peptides help regulate the body's pH levels and facilitate the removal of excess lactic acid from the muscles. This reduction in lactic acid accumulation allows athletes to maintain higher levels of intensity for longer durations without experiencing the detrimental effects of lactic acid build-up.

To understand the practical applications of these benefits, consider the example of marathon runners. Marathon runners require exceptional endurance to complete races that span over 26 miles. By incorporating peptide bioregulators into their regimen, they can enhance their aerobic capacity, allowing for more efficient oxygen use during long runs. Additionally, improved energy metabolism ensures that their muscles have a constant energy supply, reducing the risk of hitting the proverbial "wall" during the race. Furthermore, faster recovery from training sessions means they can maintain a high training volume without succumbing to fatigue, thus continuously improving their performance.

Similarly, cyclists who participate in lengthy competitions such as the Tour de France benefit from these peptides. The rigorous demands of cycling long distances at high intensities necessitate optimized oxygen delivery and utilization. Peptide bioregulators support these needs, making it possible for cyclists to sustain peak performance across multiple stages of the competition. Moreover, managing lactic acid levels becomes critical during steep climbs or sprint finishes, where anaerobic efforts are intense. Peptides that reduce lactic acid build-up enable cyclists to push harder during these pivotal moments without compromising their overall endurance.

Peptide bioregulators' influence extends to team sports as well. Sports like soccer, basketball, and rugby involve continuous movement and frequent bursts of high-intensity activity. Athletes in these sports need both endurance and the ability to recover quickly between plays. By using peptide bioregulators, they can ensure optimal energy metabolism and rapid recovery from fatigue, giving them a competitive edge on the field. Enhanced aerobic capacity also translates to better overall fitness, which is beneficial for the high-stamina demands of team-based sports.

Optimization of Training Efforts

Peptide bioregulators play a crucial role in supporting athletes' training routines by enhancing various physiological processes. One significant benefit of peptide bioregulators is their ability to promote quicker gains in strength and mass. Faster protein synthesis, stimulated by these bioregulators, directly contributes to rapid muscle growth. This means that athletes can see improvements in their physical capabilities sooner than with traditional training methods alone. The accelerated protein synthesis helps muscles repair and build more efficiently after workouts, which is essential for anyone aiming to increase their strength and muscle mass.

Maintaining a positive nitrogen balance is another critical aspect where peptide bioregulators come into play. Nitrogen is a key component of amino acids, the building blocks of proteins. For muscle tissue to grow and recover effectively, the body must retain more nitrogen than it loses. Peptide bioregulators help enhance the body's ability to maintain this positive nitrogen balance. This is particularly important for muscle recovery after intense training sessions. When athletes are able to sustain a positive nitrogen balance, they experience less muscle soreness and fatigue, allowing them to adhere to their rigorous training schedules without prolonged downtime.

The reduced risk of injury is an additional benefit provided by peptide bioregulators. Regular and intense training can place significant stress on the muscles and connective tissues, increasing the likelihood of injuries. However, optimized recovery fostered by peptide bioregulators ensures that the body heals more rapidly from the micro-damages caused by strenuous exercise. This faster healing process not only minimizes the risk of injuries but also maintains the integrity of muscles and joints over time. As a result, athletes can continue to train and compete at high levels without frequent interruptions due to injuries.

Furthermore, peptide bioregulators contribute to greater training intensity by improving nitrogen retention. When the body can better retain nitrogen, muscles have more resources available for energy production and repair. This allows athletes to push themselves harder during training sessions without experiencing early fatigue. Enhanced nitrogen retention supports prolonged periods of high-intensity exercise, enabling athletes to maximize their performance and get the most out of their workouts. Consequently, athletes can achieve significant improvements in their endurance and overall physical conditioning.

To illustrate these benefits more concretely, let's consider the example of a weightlifter. Incorporating peptide bioregulators into their regimen could lead to visible changes in muscle hypertrophy within weeks rather than months. Because protein synthesis is more efficient, the weightlifter notices increased muscle size and strength much sooner, which boosts their motivation and confidence. Additionally, maintaining a positive nitrogen balance allows the athlete to recover quickly after each lifting session, reducing the occurrence of delayed onset muscle soreness (DOMS). With less soreness, the weightlifter can train more consistently and intensively, further accelerating their progress.

Moreover, for endurance athletes such as marathon runners, peptide bioregulators can be incredibly advantageous. The improved recovery rates mean that runners experience fewer muscle strains and joint issues, which are common problems due to the repetitive nature of long-distance running. By recovering more efficiently from daily training runs, these athletes can maintain a higher mileage without risking overuse injuries. This cumulative effect of optimized recovery and sustained high training volumes ultimately leads to better race performances.

In team sports like soccer or basketball, where agility, speed, and endurance are essential, peptide bioregulators help players maintain peak performance levels throughout the season. The enhanced muscle recovery ensures that players do not suffer from chronic injuries that could sideline them for extended periods. Furthermore, the ability to train intensely without early fatigue contributes to better overall team performance, as each player can give their best effort during both practice and competition.

For those engaged in mixed-martial arts (MMA) or similar combat sports, the benefits of peptide bioregulators extend to both strength and endurance training. Faster gains in muscle mass mean fighters can reach their desired weight class more effectively while also enhancing their power and explosive strength. Improved nitrogen retention and recovery allow them to endure grueling sparring sessions and conditioning workouts without excessive fatigue. This holistic enhancement of their physical capabilities gives fighters a competitive edge, helping them perform at their best during matches.

Longevity in Athletic Career

Peptide bioregulators play an instrumental role in an athlete's long-term career longevity by preserving muscle health. This preservation is crucial as it directly impacts several aspects of an athlete's performance and overall career duration. Let's delve into how these bioregulators contribute to preserving muscle mass, maintaining consistent strength, enhancing overall performance, and offering longevity benefits.

Preserving Muscle Mass

One of the primary concerns for athletes is muscle tissue breakdown, which can occur due to strenuous training, physical stress, and aging. Peptide bioregulators can mitigate these effects by protecting muscle tissue from degeneration. These bioregulators act as signaling molecules that help regulate the body's natural processes, promoting muscle repair and growth. For instance, certain peptides have been shown to stimulate the production of growth factors essential for muscle regeneration, thereby preventing the loss of muscle mass over time.

Preserving muscle mass is vital for longevity in an athlete's career. Muscles are the engines that drive performance, and their degradation can lead to decreased strength and endurance, ultimately hampering an athlete's ability to compete at high levels. By integrating peptide bioregulators into their regimen, athletes can ensure that their muscle tissues remain robust and resilient, even under intense physical demands.

Consistent Strength Maintenance

Maintaining consistent strength is another critical aspect of an athlete's career. Fluctuations in strength can negatively impact performance during training cycles and competitions. Peptide bioregulators help stabilize these fluctuations by supporting the body's natural anabolic processes. Anabolic processes involve the synthesis of complex molecules like proteins, which are necessary for muscle building and repair.

When an athlete's body can consistently produce and repair muscle tissue, their strength levels remain stable. This stability is particularly important during long training cycles where the risk of muscle fatigue and injury is higher. For example, peptides like IGF-1 (Insulin-like Growth Factor 1) play a significant role in muscle maintenance by promoting protein synthesis and inhibiting protein breakdown. Athletes who use peptide bioregulators often report sustained strength levels, allowing them to train harder and perform better in their respective sports.

Enhanced Overall Performance

Better muscle preservation results in enhanced overall athletic performance. When muscles are healthy and well-maintained, athletes experience improved coordination, agility, and power. These improvements are not just beneficial for peak performance but also for daily training routines. Peptide bioregulators contribute to this by optimizing muscle function and reducing recovery times, enabling athletes to undergo more rigorous training with less downtime.

For instance, peptides like BPC-157 have been found to promote faster healing of muscles, tendons, and ligaments. This rapid recovery allows athletes to engage in high-intensity workouts more frequently without the risk of overtraining or injury. Moreover, preserved muscle mass means that athletes retain their explosive power and endurance, giving them a competitive edge. Whether on the field, track, or gym, the ability to maintain top-tier physical condition is a game-changer.

Longevity Benefits

The ultimate benefit of using peptide bioregulators for muscle preservation is the extension of an athlete's career. Consistent muscle health translates to fewer injuries, prolonged peak performance periods, and the ability to compete effectively for more years. Longevity in sports is not only about staying injury-free but also maintaining the physical capabilities that allow for continued success.

Athletes often face the dilemma of declining physical abilities as they age. However, those who incorporate peptide bioregulators into their health regimes can offset some of these declines. By continuously supporting muscle health, these bioregulators enable athletes to extend their competitive years, participate in more events, and achieve greater milestones. This extended career span opens up opportunities for endorsements, coaching roles, and other professional pursuits within the sports industry.

To illustrate, veteran athletes who have adopted peptide bioregulators report a noticeable difference in their physical performance and recovery as they age. They can sustain intensive training regimens without the debilitating effects of muscle wear and tear, leading to a more fulfilling and successful career. The ability to maintain high performance through advanced age not only enhances the athlete's personal achievements but also serves as inspiration for younger generations.

Gaining Competitive Edge

Peptide bioregulators have gained significant attention for their role in enhancing athletic performance. These natural compounds can provide athletes with a competitive edge, particularly by boosting stamina, maintaining peak performance, sustaining high-intensity efforts, and optimizing energy utilization.

To begin with, improved stamina is a crucial benefit that athletes can gain from peptide bioregulators. Enhanced aerobic capacity is key to boosting stamina across various sports. Aerobic capacity refers to the body's ability to deliver oxygen to muscles during prolonged physical activity. When an athlete's body efficiently delivers oxygen, it enables them to perform at higher intensities for longer periods. This capability is particularly beneficial for endurance athletes, such as marathon runners and cyclists, who rely on sustained energy output. Studies have shown that peptide bioregulators can enhance oxygen delivery and utilization in the body, thereby improving overall aerobic capacity. By increasing the efficiency of the cardiovascular system, these bioregulators help athletes maintain high levels of stamina throughout their training and competitions.

Another critical advantage offered by peptide bioregulators is peak performance maintenance. Athletes often face the challenge of recovering quickly from fatigue to maintain peak performance during sustained activities. Peptide bioregulators facilitate quicker recovery by promoting muscle repair and reducing inflammation. For instance, after intense training sessions or competitive events, muscles can become fatigued due to micro-tears in muscle fibers. Bioregulators support the body's natural healing processes, ensuring that athletes recover faster and are ready for the next challenge. This ability to bounce back swiftly is particularly important for sports that involve repeated bouts of activity with minimal rest, such as soccer, basketball, and tennis. By aiding rapid recovery, peptide bioregulators help athletes sustain their peak performance levels without compromising their overall training regimen.

In addition to maintaining peak performance, peptide bioregulators play a vital role in sustaining high-intensity effort. One of the primary limitations to prolonged high-intensity performance is the build-up of lactic acid in muscles. Lactic acid is a byproduct of anaerobic metabolism, and its accumulation can lead to muscle cramps, fatigue, and decreased performance. Peptide bioregulators can help manage and reduce lactic acid build-up, allowing athletes to continue performing at high intensity for extended periods. This benefit is especially valuable for athletes involved in high-intensity interval training (HIIT), sprinting, weightlifting, and other activities that require short bursts of maximal effort. By lowering lactic acid levels, bioregulators enable athletes to push their limits and achieve new performance milestones.

Enhanced energy utilization is another significant benefit provided by peptide bioregulators. Efficient energy metabolism is critical for prolonged exertion during competitions. The body's ability to metabolize energy efficiently determines how long athletes can sustain their performance before reaching exhaustion. Peptide bioregulators optimize energy metabolism by increasing the efficiency of mitochondrial function—the powerhouse of cells where energy production occurs. With improved mitochondrial efficiency, athletes can generate more energy from the same amount of fuel, be it carbohydrates, fats, or proteins. This optimization ensures that athletes have a steady supply of energy throughout their activities, reducing the likelihood of hitting the proverbial "wall" during long-distance events or grueling matches.

Furthermore, peptide bioregulators contribute to overall better health and reduced stress on the body, which indirectly benefits athletic performance. By supporting various physiological functions, including immune response and hormonal balance, bioregulators create a more resilient body capable of enduring the rigors of intense training and competition. A well-functioning immune system means fewer illnesses and disruptions to training schedules, while hormonal balance supports optimal muscle growth and repair.

To illustrate these points, consider the example of an elite triathlete who undergoes rigorous training involving swimming, cycling, and running. This athlete would benefit from improved stamina through enhanced aerobic capacity, enabling them to maintain a strong pace during each segment of the triathlon. During recovery phases between training sessions or races, peptide bioregulators would aid in quicker muscle repair, allowing the athlete to train consistently without the setback of prolonged fatigue. During high-intensity segments, such as sprint finishes or uphill climbs, reduced lactic acid build-up would ensure sustained performance, keeping the athlete in competitive form. Finally, enhanced energy utilization would provide the necessary fuel efficiency for the athlete to perform optimally throughout the event, minimizing energy wastage and delaying the onset of fatigue.

This chapter delved into the significant ways peptide bioregulators can enhance athletic performance naturally by promoting muscle growth and improving endurance. We examined how these peptides boost protein synthesis, retain nitrogen, and accelerate recovery processes. These functions work together to facilitate quicker and more effective muscle development, allowing athletes to maximize their strength and minimize recovery time. By inhibiting muscle breakdown, peptide bioregulators also help maintain and protect the gains made during training.

Furthermore, we explored how peptide bioregulators can improve stamina and energy utilization, vital for sustained athletic performance. By increasing aerobic capacity and promoting efficient energy metabolism, these peptides enable athletes to perform at higher intensities for longer periods. Enhanced oxygen delivery and reduced lactic acid build-up contribute to prolonged endurance and faster recovery from fatigue. Together, these benefits illustrate the comprehensive impact of peptide bioregulators on both muscle growth and overall athletic performance, making them a valuable addition to an athlete's regimen.

CHAPTER 5

Cognitive Health and Brain Boost

E nhancing cognitive health and boosting brain function are essential for maintaining a high quality of life, especially in today's fast-paced world. This chapter delves into the intriguing realm of peptide bioregulators, molecules that hold significant promise for improving various aspects of cognitive performance. These small but powerful protein fragments have been shown to enhance memory, focus, and concentration by interacting with neural pathways and promoting brain health. Peptide bioregulators offer an exciting avenue for those seeking to optimize their mental capabilities and achieve better cognitive resilience.

Throughout this chapter, we will explore how peptide bioregulators can target neural mechanisms to support memory enhancement, spotlighting their role in neuroplasticity, synaptic plasticity, and oxidative stress mitigation. We will also examine their impact on focus and concentration by addressing mental clarity, stress reduction, neurotransmitter balance, and neuroprotection. Furthermore, the discussion extends to the peptides' ability to activate neuroplasticity and support synaptic health, which are crucial for long-term brain function and adaptability. This comprehensive examination provides readers with evidence-based insights into how these molecules can be integrated into a holistic approach to cognitive health, ultimately contributing to improved mental performance and longevity.

Memory Enhancement

Peptide bioregulators have gained attention for their potential to enhance memory by targeting neural pathways and promoting neurogenesis. These small protein fragments are designed to influence various biological processes, particularly in the brain, where they can support cognitive function in multiple ways.

One of the key mechanisms through which peptide bioregulators support memory improvement is by enhancing neuroplasticity. Neuroplasticity refers to the brain's ability to reorganize itself by forming new neural connections throughout one's life. This capacity is crucial for learning and retaining new information. Peptide bioregulators play a vital role in this process by providing the necessary environment for neurons to create and strengthen synapses. This enhanced connectivity allows for better communication between different parts of the brain, facilitating learning and information retention.

Moreover, these peptides facilitate communication between neurons, thereby improving synaptic plasticity. Synaptic plasticity is essential for efficient information processing and recall. It involves the strengthening or weakening of synapses, depending on the level of activity. By promoting synaptic plasticity, peptide bioregulators ensure that the brain is more adaptable and capable of handling complex tasks. This adaptability is particularly beneficial for memory formation and retrieval, as it allows the brain to store and access information more efficiently.

In addition to their role in enhancing neuroplasticity and synaptic communication, peptide bioregulators also help mitigate oxidative stress in the brain. Oxidative stress occurs when there is an imbalance between free radicals and antioxidants in the body, leading to cellular damage. In the brain, oxidative stress is closely linked to memory decline and cognitive impairment. Peptide bioregulators contribute to reducing oxidative stress by promoting the activity of antioxidants, which neutralize free radicals and protect brain cells from damage. This protective effect helps preserve cognitive function and prevent memory deterioration.

Furthermore, peptide bioregulators may promote the production of brain-derived neurotrophic factor (BDNF), a protein that plays a critical role in neurogenesis and synaptic plasticity. BDNF is essential for the growth and maintenance of neurons, as well as for long-term memory formation. By increasing the levels of BDNF in the brain, peptide bioregulators can enhance cognitive performance and memory retention. This boost in BDNF production supports the brain's ability to adapt to new information and experiences, ultimately leading to improved mental performance.

To maximize the benefits of peptide bioregulators, it is important to incorporate them into a comprehensive cognitive health strategy. This includes maintaining a balanced diet rich in antioxidants, engaging in regular physical exercise, and practicing mental exercises that challenge the brain. Combining these lifestyle choices with the use of peptide bioregulators can create a synergistic effect, amplifying the positive impact on memory and overall cognitive function.

Increasing Focus and Concentration

Peptide bioregulators are becoming increasingly recognized for their potential to enhance cognitive function, particularly in the realms of focus and concentration. These small molecules work by interacting with the body's natural biological processes, thereby promoting mental clarity and boosting brain health. This subpoint will delve into the mechanisms through which peptide bioregulators operate and their practical applications in enhancing decision-making, reducing stress, balancing neurotransmitters, and offering neuroprotective benefits.

One of the primary ways in which peptide bioregulators improve focus and concentration is by promoting mental clarity. Mental clarity is crucial for effective decision-making and productivity. In a fast-paced world, the ability to think clearly and make informed decisions quickly can make a significant difference in both personal and professional settings. Peptide bioregulators achieve this by optimizing the function of neurons and supporting neural pathways. When these pathways are functioning efficiently, the communication between neurons is enhanced, leading to streamlined thought processes and heightened awareness. This improved mental clarity allows individuals to process information more effectively, leading to better decision-making capabilities and increased productivity.

Another significant benefit of peptide bioregulators is their ability to modulate stress responses. Stress is a common barrier to maintaining focus and concentration. High-stress levels can lead to mental fatigue, decreased attention span, and overall cognitive decline. Peptide bioregulators help mitigate these effects by interacting with the stress response system of the body. They regulate the production of stress hormones such as cortisol, thereby reducing stress levels. Lower stress levels result in enhanced attention and mental stamina, allowing individuals to maintain focus for extended periods. By incorporating peptides into their routine, individuals may experience a more balanced and stable emotional state, which contributes to sustained cognitive performance.

Guideline: To effectively manage stress with peptide bioregulators, it is essential to integrate them with other stress-reduction techniques such as mindfulness, adequate sleep, and regular physical exercise. Combining these approaches can lead to optimal results in reducing stress and improving cognitive performance.

Supporting neurotransmitter balance is another avenue through which peptide bioregulators enhance focus and concentration. Neurotransmitters are chemical messengers that transmit signals between neurons. An imbalance in these chemicals can lead to sluggish cognitive function and impaired information processing. Peptide bioregulators help maintain the equilibrium of neurotransmitters such as dopamine, serotonin, and acetylcholine, which are vital for mood regulation, alertness, and cognitive speed. By ensuring that these neurotransmitters are in balance, peptides contribute to faster decision-making and problem-solving abilities. The enhanced processing speed not only improves focus but also supports overall cognitive efficiency.

Guideline: Balancing neurotransmitters can be augmented by consuming a diet rich in essential nutrients such as omega-3 fatty acids, B vitamins, and amino acids, which support the production and function of neurotransmitters. Complementing peptide supplementation with a nutrient-dense diet can further enhance cognitive health.

The neuroprotective properties of peptide bioregulators play a critical role in sustaining long-term brain health. Neuroprotection involves safeguarding neurons from damage and degeneration, which is essential for preserving cognitive functions like focus and concentration over time. Peptides protect against various neurotoxic factors, including oxidative stress and inflammation, which are known to impair brain function. By mitigating these harmful effects, peptide bioregulators help maintain the integrity of neuronal structures and functions, ensuring that the brain remains healthy and capable of performing optimally even as one ages.

Guideline: For comprehensive brain protection, consider adopting a holistic approach that includes regular physical activity, intellectual stimulation, and a balanced diet, alongside peptide supplementation. These combined strategies create a synergistic effect that promotes enduring brain health and cognitive vitality.

Neuroplasticity Activation

How Peptide Bioregulators Activate Neuroplasticity to Support Cognitive Function

Neuroplasticity is the brain's remarkable ability to reorganize itself by forming new neural connections throughout life. This capacity is essential for learning new skills, adapting to changes, and recovering from injuries. Peptide bioregulators have garnered interest for their potential to activate neuroplasticity, thereby supporting cognitive function.

The concept of neuroplasticity serves as the cornerstone of our understanding of how learning and memory operate. When we learn a new skill or absorb new information, our brains undergo structural and functional changes. Neural connections become stronger or weaker depending on our experiences, ultimately shaping our capabilities and behavior. By harnessing this natural process, peptide bioregulators can enhance learning and memory retention.

One area where enhanced neuroplasticity shows profound effects is in memory retention. Studies have indicated that a more plastic brain has better memory retention capabilities. This means that individuals can recall past experiences and learned skills more effectively when their brains are more adaptable. Enhanced neuroplasticity ensures that neurons communicate more efficiently, making it easier to store and retrieve information. As a result, cognitive health improves, reducing the risk of age-related cognitive decline and other neurological disorders.

A dynamic brain environment, characterized by continuous formation and modification of neural pathways, is crucial for optimal aging and cognitive resilience. Over time, our brains can naturally lose some of their plasticity; however, maintaining high levels of neuroplasticity can help mitigate these effects. A more adaptable brain is better equipped to handle the challenges of aging, including memory loss and diminished cognitive function.

Peptide bioregulators play a vital role in maintaining and enhancing neuroplasticity. These molecules work at a cellular level, influencing gene expression and protein synthesis, which are critical for neural growth and repair. By targeting specific pathways in the brain, peptide bioregulators can stimulate the production of brain-derived neurotrophic factor (BDNF) and other neurotrophins. BDNF is known to support neuron survival, growth, and the formation of synaptic connections, all of which are essential for healthy brain function.

To foster neuroplasticity through targeted peptide supplementation, consider incorporating the following actionable steps into your wellness routine:

1. **Consult a Healthcare Professional** : Before beginning any new supplement regimen, it's important to consult with a healthcare provider who can offer personalized advice and monitor your progress.
1. **Choose High-Quality Supplements** : Not all peptide supplements are created equal. Look for reputable brands that provide transparency about their ingredients and manufacturing processes.
1. **Follow Recommended Dosages** : Adhering to the suggested dosage guidelines is crucial for achieving desired results without adverse effects.
1. **Combine with a Balanced Diet** : A diet rich in antioxidants, omega-3 fatty acids, and vitamins can complement peptide supplementation by providing essential nutrients for brain health.
1. **Engage in Continuous Learning** : Regularly challenging your brain with new activities such as puzzles, reading, and learning new skills can help maintain its plasticity.
1. **Exercise Regularly** : Physical activity has been shown to increase BDNF levels and promote neuroplasticity. Aim for at least 30 minutes of moderate exercise most days of the week.
1. **Manage Stress** : Chronic stress can impair neuroplasticity. Practice stress-reducing techniques like meditation, deep breathing exercises, or yoga to keep your mind calm and focused.
1. **Get Enough Sleep** : Quality sleep is essential for brain health and neuroplasticity. Strive for 7-9 hours of sleep per night to ensure your brain has adequate time to repair and regenerate.

By following these steps, you can create an environment that supports and enhances neuroplasticity, thereby improving cognitive function and overall brain health. It's important to recognize that while peptide bioregulators offer promising benefits, they should be part of a holistic approach to brain health that includes lifestyle modifications and regular monitoring by healthcare professionals.

Stress Reduction

Peptide bioregulators offer a promising avenue for improving cognitive performance by reducing stress levels. Understanding the intricate relationship between stress and cognitive function is key to appreciating how these molecules can be leveraged for mental enhancement.

Low stress levels are fundamental to maintaining focus, concentration, and overall mental stamina. Stress, whether acute or chronic, diverts cognitive resources away from tasks that require deep thinking and prolonged attention. When stress levels are high, the brain operates in a state of heightened alertness, leading to quicker fatigue and diminished capacity for sustained concentration. By reducing stress, peptide bioregulators help create an internal environment where the brain can perform optimally, free from the distraction and weariness caused by stress-induced states.

Moreover, the reduction of stress leads to better cognitive clarity, which significantly improves everyday decision-making and productivity. Cognitive clarity refers to the sharpness and lucidity of thought processes, enabling individuals to make more informed and effective decisions. When stress is minimized, the mind is clearer and more adept at evaluating options and outcomes. This clarity streamlines the cognitive load, making it easier to process information and arrive at sound conclusions promptly. In professional settings, this translates to enhanced productivity as tasks are completed more efficiently and with greater precision.

To maximize the benefits of stress reduction on cognitive performance, integrating stress management techniques with peptide use is essential. Strategies such as mindfulness meditation, physical exercise, and adequate sleep play crucial roles in managing stress. Mindfulness meditation, for instance, has been shown to reduce cortisol levels, a primary stress hormone, thereby contributing to lower overall stress. Regular physical exercise not only helps in managing stress but also promotes the release of endorphins, which further aid in mood regulation. Additionally, ensuring adequate sleep is vital, as lack of sleep exacerbates stress and impairs cognitive functions such as memory and executive function. Combining these stress management practices with the targeted use of peptide bioregulators creates a comprehensive approach to sustaining low-stress levels and enhancing cognitive performance.

Addressing stress is essential for sustained cognitive health and mental well-being. Prolonged stress exposure has detrimental effects on the brain, including shrinkage of the prefrontal cortex (the area responsible for decision-making and executive functions) and enlargement of the amygdala (the region involved in emotional responses). These changes can lead to impaired cognitive abilities, increased anxiety, and difficulty handling complex tasks. By utilizing peptide bioregulators to manage and reduce stress, individuals protect their brains from these harmful structural changes, preserving cognitive functions and promoting long-term mental health.

Exploring the mechanisms by which peptide bioregulators achieve stress reduction offers deeper insights into their efficacy. Peptide bioregulators work by modulating specific biological pathways that govern stress responses. For example, certain peptides influence the hypothalamic-pituitary-adrenal (HPA) axis, which plays a critical role in the body's reaction to stress. By regulating the HPA axis, these peptides help to maintain hormonal balance, preventing excessive release of stress hormones like cortisol. This hormonal equilibrium supports a calmer, more focused state of mind conducive to optimal cognitive functioning.

In addition to hormonal regulation, peptide bioregulators may also affect neurotransmitter systems involved in mood and cognition. Neurotransmitters such as serotonin and dopamine are pivotal in mood regulation and cognitive processes. Peptides that enhance the availability or efficiency of these neurotransmitters can alleviate stress and elevate mood, thereby indirectly supporting better cognitive performance. For instance, peptides that increase serotonin levels promote feelings of well-being and relaxation, reducing stress and fostering an environment where cognitive tasks can be performed with greater ease and effectiveness.

Furthermore, peptide bioregulators might have antioxidant properties that protect the brain from oxidative stress, another contributor to cognitive decline. Oxidative stress results from an imbalance between free radicals and antioxidants in the body, leading to cellular damage. The brain, being highly metabolically active, is particularly susceptible to oxidative stress, which can impair neuronal function and accelerate cognitive aging. By mitigating oxidative stress, peptides safeguard neuronal integrity and support sustained cognitive abilities throughout life.

Considering practical applications of peptide bioregulators for stress management, it is pertinent to discuss dosage, timing, and combination with other supplements or lifestyle practices. Appropriate dosing is crucial to achieving desired outcomes without adverse effects. Consulting healthcare providers for personalized recommendations ensures safe and effective peptide use. Timing also plays a role; for instance, some peptides may be more beneficial when taken in the morning to support daily cognitive demands, while others might be better suited for evening use to promote relaxation and restful sleep.

Combining peptides with other natural supplements known for their stress-relieving properties, such as adaptogenic herbs (e.g., ashwagandha, rhodiola), can provide synergistic effects. Adaptogens help the body adapt to stressors and normalize physiological functions, complementing the actions of peptide bioregulators. A holistic approach incorporating diet, exercise, mindfulness practices, and appropriate supplementation offers a robust framework for managing stress and harnessing its cognitive benefits.

Supporting Synaptic Health

Peptide bioregulators play a crucial role in supporting synaptic health, which significantly enhances cognitive functions. Synapses are the points of communication between neurons, where neurotransmitters transmit signals that allow our brain to process information. Improved synaptic communication is vital for efficient information processing and recall, contributing to better memory and overall mental clarity.

Firstly, the importance of synaptic communication cannot be overstated. It is the foundation of how our brain processes and stores information. When synapses function optimally, the transmission of signals between neurons becomes more efficient, leading to faster and more accurate information processing. This efficiency is essential for carrying out everyday tasks that require quick thinking and decision-making. In essence, healthy synaptic communication ensures that our brains are operating at peak performance.

There is a direct relationship between synaptic health and memory strength. Memory formation and retrieval depend heavily on the quality of synaptic connections. Peptides, small chains of amino acids, enhance synaptic health by promoting the creation and maintenance of these connections. As peptides support synaptic plasticity—the ability of synapses to strengthen or weaken over time—they play a critical role in cognitive enhancement. This means that individuals using peptide bioregulators may experience improved memory retention and recall, making it easier to remember important information and learn new things.

One example of a peptide that supports synaptic health is Cerebrolysin. This peptide has been shown to improve cognitive function in various studies. For instance, research indicates that Cerebrolysin can enhance memory and learning capabilities by promoting neuronal survival and growth. By boosting the health of synaptic connections, peptides like Cerebrolysin provide a tangible benefit to cognitive performance.

Additionally, peptides protect against oxidative stress, which is a significant factor in cognitive decline. Oxidative stress occurs when there is an imbalance between free radicals and antioxidants in the body, leading to damage of cells and tissues, including those in the brain. Peptides have antioxidant properties that help neutralize free radicals, reducing oxidative damage. By preserving the integrity of brain structures involved in memory and cognition, peptides contribute to long-term cognitive health.

For example, the peptide Epithalon is known for its potent antioxidant effects. Studies have shown that Epithalon can reduce markers of oxidative stress in the brain, thereby protecting neurons from damage. This protection is crucial for maintaining synaptic health and ensuring that cognitive functions remain sharp as we age.

The synergy between healthy synapses and overall cognitive resilience is another key aspect of how peptide bioregulators support brain health. Cognitive resilience refers to the brain's ability to adapt and function well despite challenges such as aging or stressful environments. Healthy synapses provide the stable foundation needed for this resilience, allowing the brain to recover and adapt more effectively. By enhancing synaptic health, peptides not only boost immediate cognitive functions but also contribute to the brain's long-term adaptability and robustness.

To illustrate this point further, consider the peptide Semax. Semax has been shown to influence neuroplasticity, the brain's ability to reorganize itself by forming new neural connections. This capability is essential for learning and adapting to new situations. By promoting neuroplasticity, Semax helps maintain cognitive resilience, ensuring that the brain remains flexible and capable of handling various cognitive demands.

Moreover, the benefits of peptide bioregulators extend beyond just supporting synaptic health. They also play a role in modulating neurotransmitter levels, which are critical for mood regulation and overall cognitive function. Balanced neurotransmitter levels ensure that synaptic communication occurs smoothly, preventing issues such as depression or anxiety that can hinder cognitive performance. For instance, the peptide Selank has been found to balance GABA and serotonin levels in the brain, promoting a calm and focused mental state conducive to optimal cognitive function.

These combined actions of peptides—enhancing synaptic health, protecting against oxidative stress, and balancing neurotransmitter levels—create a holistic approach to improving cognitive performance. Individuals who incorporate peptide bioregulators into their wellness routines may find that they experience greater mental clarity, enhanced memory, and improved focus. This holistic improvement is particularly beneficial for busy professionals who need to maintain high levels of focus and productivity, as well as for athletes seeking to optimize their mental and physical performance.

This chapter has detailed the potential benefits of peptide bioregulators in enhancing cognitive functions such as memory, focus, and concentration. By supporting neuroplasticity and synaptic communication, these molecules can create an optimal environment for brain health. The chapter also discussed how peptide bioregulators help mitigate oxidative stress, promote the production of brain-derived neurotrophic factor (BDNF), and balance neurotransmitter levels, all contributing to improved mental clarity and performance.

In addition, the chapter highlighted practical applications for integrating peptide bioregulators into a cognitive health strategy. Combining these supplements with a balanced diet rich in antioxidants, regular physical exercise, and mental exercises can amplify their positive effects on brain function. By doing so, individuals may experience enhanced memory retention, better decision-making skills, and overall cognitive vitality, ultimately supporting their quest for improved mental performance and longevity.

CHAPTER 6

Practical Applications: Delivery Methods

Incorporating peptide bioregulators into daily routines can be achieved through various practical methods. By leveraging these techniques, individuals can enhance their wellness regimen with ease and efficiency. This chapter aims to provide a comprehensive overview of two primary delivery methods: oral supplements and topical applications.

Readers will find detailed discussions on the different forms of oral supplements, such as capsules, powders, and liquids, explaining their unique benefits and how they cater to specific health needs. Additionally, the chapter explores the array of topical products available, including creams, gels, and serums. The focus will be on understanding which form works best for different skin types and goals, ensuring readers have the tools to make informed choices in integrating peptide bioregulators into their lifestyles.

Types of Oral Supplements

When it comes to incorporating peptide bioregulators into daily routines, oral supplements offer a range of practical and efficient options. Here, we delve into the specifics of three main forms: capsules, powders, and liquids, each providing unique advantages tailored to different needs and preferences.

One of the most popular forms of oral peptide bioregulators is capsules. Capsules are convenient and easy to consume, making them an excellent choice for individuals seeking simplicity in their supplement regimen. The encapsulated peptides come in pre-measured doses, ensuring that users can easily take the correct amount without the need for measuring spoons or scales. This precision in dosing is particularly beneficial for those who wish to adhere strictly to their supplementation plan. Moreover, capsules are portable, allowing individuals to maintain their supplement routine even when on the go. Whether traveling for work or leisure, carrying a small bottle of capsules is hassle-free. The ease of consumption also appeals to busy professionals and those with tight schedules, as it takes only a moment to swallow a capsule with water, integrating seamlessly into any lifestyle.

In addition to their convenience, capsules protect the peptides from the harsh environment of the stomach. The encasing material often ensures that the peptides are only released once they reach the intestine, where absorption occurs more effectively. This protection helps maintain the efficacy of the peptides, allowing users to experience the full benefits. For health enthusiasts and individuals focused on anti-aging solutions, this means maximizing the potential of their chosen supplements without worrying about degradation during digestion.

Another form of oral peptide bioregulators gaining popularity is powder. Powders are highly versatile, offering flexibility in how they are consumed. Users can mix the powder with various beverages, such as water, juice, or smoothies, creating a customized intake experience. This versatility makes powders an appealing option for athletes and fitness aficionados who might already incorporate shakes into their workout routines. Adding peptide bioregulator powder to their drinks can be a simple way to enhance muscle growth, recovery times, and overall performance. Furthermore, powders allow for adjustable dosing. Individuals can easily measure and tweak the amount of powder they use based on their specific health goals and responses to the supplement. This adaptability is particularly valuable for those engaged in intensive fitness programs or training regimens, as it allows them to tailor their supplementation precisely to their evolving needs.

For those concerned about cognitive decline or looking to boost mental clarity and focus, peptide powders can be incorporated into morning routines alongside other nootropic beverages. Mixing the powder into coffee or tea provides an effortless way to start the day with an added cognitive edge. The ability to blend powders into different drinks not only enhances the user experience but also encourages consistent use, as individuals can integrate them into their favorite daily beverages without altering their habits significantly.

Liquids represent another effective form of oral peptide bioregulators, known for their fast absorption rates. Liquid supplements are ideal for anyone who has difficulty swallowing pills or simply prefers an alternative to solid forms. The liquid form ensures that the peptides are quickly absorbed into the bloodstream, often leading to faster onset of effects. This rapid absorption is particularly beneficial for individuals seeking immediate benefits, such as improved energy levels or quicker recovery post-exercise. Liquid peptides can be taken directly using a dropper or mixed into beverages, providing a flexible administration method. This flexibility is especially useful for holistic health enthusiasts who prefer to avoid synthetic additives and stick to natural, straightforward supplement forms. Additionally, liquids can be easily incorporated into existing health routines, such as mixing them into herbal teas or fresh juices, aligning with broader wellness strategies.

The quick absorption of liquid peptide bioregulators means that users may notice improvements sooner, enhancing adherence and satisfaction with the supplement regimen. This immediacy can be motivating, encouraging continued use and fostering long-term commitment to health and wellness goals. For busy professionals, the fast-acting nature of liquid peptides can provide the support needed to maintain focus and productivity throughout demanding days. Similarly, athletes may find that the prompt onset of benefits aids in rapid recovery and sustained performance.

Dosing Guidelines for Oral Supplements

Practical Applications: Delivery Methods

When it comes to incorporating peptide bioregulators into your daily routine, understanding the correct dosage is crucial. Getting the right amount can maximize benefits and help you achieve your health goals more effectively. Here are some recommendations and guidelines tailored to help you determine the optimal dosage based on individual health objectives.

Individual Health Goals

First and foremost, it's essential to establish your specific health goals. Whether you aim to improve athletic performance, enhance cognitive function, support anti-aging efforts, or boost overall well-being, each objective can influence the recommended dosage of peptide bioregulators. For example, athletes looking to enhance muscle growth might need a higher dose compared to someone focusing on cognitive enhancement.

Athletes and fitness enthusiasts should consider dosages that support muscle repair and recovery. A typical recommendation could range from 1-2 milligrams per kilogram of body weight per day for muscle growth and recovery. In contrast, those interested in anti-aging and wellness may benefit from lower doses, such as 0.5-1 milligram per kilogram of body weight daily, focusing more on longevity and cellular repair.

Those concerned about cognitive decline might find that dosages tailored to improve mental clarity and memory are beneficial. Such individuals might start with a baseline of 1 milligram per kilogram of body weight daily and adjust according to how they respond over time. This perspective allows flexibility in tailoring the dosage to meet unique cognitive needs.

For holistic health enthusiasts, including those exploring alternative medicine and wellness supplements, a balanced approach is ideal. Depending on their objectives—whether it's improving skin health, boosting immunity, or enhancing vitality—their dosages might vary but generally fall within a moderate range, ensuring balanced and holistic benefits without overwhelming the system.

Adherence to Dosages

Adhering to recommended dosages is paramount to avoid potential complications. Overdosing can lead to adverse effects, diminishing the very benefits you're seeking. Each individual's body responds differently to peptides, and sticking to the prescribed amounts helps maintain a safe and effective regimen.

Consistency also plays a key role. Taking your supplements at the same time each day ensures steady levels of peptides in your system, contributing to sustained benefits. Mark your calendar or set reminders to keep track of your intake schedule, making it easier to stick to the routine without missing any doses.

Dosage Adjustment

An important consideration when using peptide bioregulators is the ability to adjust dosages based on personal experience and evolving health needs. As you begin your journey, starting with a lower dose is often advisable. This conservative approach allows you to monitor how your body responds, minimizing risks while gathering insights on effectiveness.

After an initial period, typically a few weeks, you can evaluate how well the current dosage is meeting your health goals. Keep a journal noting any changes in your physical and mental well-being, performance metrics, or overall vitality. If improvements are noted, you might decide to maintain the current dosage. However, if results are not aligning with expectations, gradual adjustments can be made.

For instance, if you're not seeing expected improvements in muscle recovery as an athlete, you might increase the dosage incrementally by 0.5 milligrams per kilogram of body weight and observe the outcomes over another few weeks. Conversely, if experiencing side effects such as digestive discomfort, reducing the dosage slightly may alleviate these issues while still providing benefits.

It's also valuable to listen to your body's cues. Fatigue, insomnia, or other unusual symptoms can indicate that modifications are needed. Flexibility and attentiveness in adjusting doses ensure you stay on track toward achieving desired health outcomes.

Professional Consultation

While self-monitoring and adjustment are useful, consulting healthcare professionals is highly recommended for personalized advice and safety. Healthcare providers can offer customized recommendations tailored to your specific conditions, needs, and goals. They can conduct necessary tests and assessments to determine optimal dosages and monitor your progress scientifically.

Professional guidance becomes even more crucial if you have underlying health conditions or are taking other medications. Interactions between peptide bioregulators and other treatments need careful evaluation to prevent adverse effects. Your healthcare provider can integrate peptide use into your broader health plan, ensuring all elements work synergistically.

Involving professionals also enhances the effectiveness of your peptide regimen. With access to the latest research and medical insights, practitioners can provide evidence-based recommendations, optimizing both dosage and delivery methods.

Additionally, regular follow-ups with your healthcare provider allow for ongoing adjustments and refinements. As your health evolves, so too can your peptide bioregulator strategy, ensuring continuous alignment with your goals.

Summary

Timing of Intake for Oral Supplements

Timing is a crucial factor when it comes to taking oral supplements, as it can significantly affect their efficacy and overall benefits. Understanding the optimal times for consumption, the relationship between supplements and meals, establishing a routine, and maximizing absorption through timed intake are all key components to ensure that one gets the most out of their supplementation regimen.

Ideal Consumption Times: The timing of supplement intake can greatly influence how well the body absorbs and utilizes these nutrients. For many supplements, taking them at specific times of the day can enhance their effectiveness. For instance, vitamins that support energy production, such as B vitamins, are often best taken in the morning. This timing aligns with the body's natural rhythm and can help boost energy levels throughout the day. On the other hand, supplements like magnesium, which promote relaxation and sleep, are typically recommended for evening use. Similarly, fat-soluble vitamins (A, D, E, and K) are better absorbed when taken with meals containing dietary fats, whereas water-soluble vitamins (like vitamin C and B-complex) can be taken on an empty stomach or with food.

When it comes to protein supplements, athletes and fitness enthusiasts might find it beneficial to consume them shortly after workouts. This practice helps in muscle recovery and growth by providing the necessary amino acids at a time when the muscles are more receptive to nutrient uptake. Furthermore, some cognitive-enhancing supplements, often referred to as nootropics, are best taken in the morning to support mental clarity and focus throughout the day. Adhering to these ideal consumption times ensures that the body receives the maximum benefit from each type of supplement.

Meal Association: Another important aspect to consider is whether supplements should be taken with or without food. This largely depends on the specific supplement and its interaction with various nutrients in food. Some supplements are better absorbed when taken with a meal because they require certain substances found in food to facilitate absorption. For example, taking iron supplements with a source of vitamin C (like an orange or bell pepper) can significantly enhance iron absorption. Conversely, calcium can hinder the absorption of iron, so it's advisable not to take these two minerals together.

However, there are also supplements that may cause gastrointestinal discomfort if taken on an empty stomach. Fish oil supplements, which are rich in omega-3 fatty acids, can sometimes lead to burping or indigestion if consumed without food. To avoid such unpleasant effects, it's generally recommended to take these supplements with meals. Additionally, probiotics, which help maintain gut health, are typically advised to be taken either with food or just before a meal to maximize their survival through the acidic environment of the stomach and reach the intestines where they exert their beneficial effects. Understanding meal association can make supplement intake more comfortable and efficient.

Routine Creation: Establishing a consistent supplement intake routine is vital for maintaining compliance and ensuring that the body receives nutrients regularly. One practical way to create a routine is by associating supplement intake with daily habits. For instance, placing supplements near items you use every morning, like your toothbrush or coffee maker, can serve as a visual reminder. Setting alarms or using smartphone apps designed to track supplement intake can also help keep consistency on track.

It's also important to start slow and gradually build up the routine. Begin with one or two supplements and once the habit is established, add more as needed. Spacing out supplements throughout the day can prevent overwhelming the digestive system and ensure that the body has a steady supply of nutrients. Consistency is particularly important for supplements that require regular intake to build up in the body, such as vitamin D or magnesium. Over time, a routine can become second nature, much like brushing teeth or having meals, thus making it easier to remember and sustain long-term.

Absorption Maximization: Maximizing absorption through timed consumption can further enhance the effectiveness of supplements. Certain nutrients have specific windows during which they are best absorbed. For example, calcium is better absorbed in smaller doses spread throughout the day rather than a single large dose. This approach takes advantage of the body's ability to absorb calcium more efficiently in smaller amounts.

Another strategy involves understanding the body's circadian rhythms, which are natural physiological cycles that repeat roughly every 24 hours. Aligning supplement intake with these cycles can optimize absorption and utilization. For example, studies have shown that the body's absorption of calcium is better during the evening, making it beneficial to take calcium supplements at night. Moreover, nutrients like collagen, which support skin health and joint function, are often taken before bedtime since the body undergoes repair and regeneration processes during sleep.

Hydration also plays a critical role in nutrient absorption. Ensuring adequate water intake throughout the day can aid in the digestion and assimilation of supplements. However, it's essential to strike a balance as excessive water intake at the time of supplement consumption can dilute digestive enzymes and hinder absorption. Therefore, drinking a moderate amount of water with supplements is generally recommended.

In addition to hydration, combining certain supplements with complementary nutrients can enhance absorption. For instance, pairing vitamin D with calcium supplements can boost calcium absorption as vitamin D facilitates the transport of calcium into the bloodstream. Similarly, taking omega-3 supplements alongside fat-soluble vitamins can improve the bioavailability of these nutrients.

Forms of Topical Products

Topical peptide products have gained popularity due to their diverse benefits and effective delivery methods. Understanding the different forms these products can take, as well as their specific benefits, allows individuals to make informed choices tailored to their skin needs.

One of the most common forms of topical peptide products is creams. Creams are typically rich in moisturizing agents, making them ideal for providing hydration to the skin. The cream's consistency allows for a prolonged release of active ingredients over time. This means that peptides are gradually delivered to the skin, ensuring sustained hydration and longer-lasting effects. For those dealing with dry or mature skin, which often requires more intensive moisture, creams can be a particularly beneficial option. Hydrated skin not only looks healthier but also improves the absorption and efficacy of the peptides themselves.

In addition to creams, gels are another form of topical peptide products. Gels offer faster absorption compared to creams, which can be advantageous for individuals with oily or combination skin types. The lightweight texture of gels ensures that active ingredients penetrate quickly, leaving behind no greasy residue. This quick absorption helps reduce the likelihood of clogged pores, making gels suitable for acne-prone skin as well. The fast-acting nature of gels can provide immediate hydration and peptide benefits without the heaviness that some moisturizers might bring. For fitness enthusiasts who may experience oilier skin due to sweat and frequent workouts, gels offer a refreshing and efficient skincare solution.

Serums are yet another form through which peptides can be applied topically. Serums are known for their concentrated formulations, which are designed to deliver targeted results. These potent elixirs often contain higher concentrations of active ingredients than creams or gels. This makes serums especially useful for addressing specific skin concerns such as fine lines, wrinkles, or hyperpigmentation. Due to their lightweight consistency, serums can penetrate deeply into the skin, allowing peptides to reach the layers where they can be most effective. Individuals looking to tackle particular aging signs or skin damage will find serums to be a powerful tool in their skincare arsenals.

Choosing the right formulation of topical peptide products is crucial and should be based on individual skin types and conditions. Each skin type has specific needs that can be addressed more effectively with the correct product form. For instance, someone with dry, flaky skin would benefit more from a hydrating cream, while an individual with oily skin would likely find better results with a lightweight gel. Furthermore, understanding one's skin condition—whether it is prone to acne, sensitivity, or pigmentation issues—can guide the selection of the most appropriate peptide product. It's always beneficial to perform a patch test before fully incorporating any new product into a daily skincare routine. This helps avoid potential adverse reactions and ensures that the product aligns well with one's unique skin properties.

For people interested in anti-aging solutions, the different forms of topical peptide products offer tailored approaches. Peptide creams, with their hydrating benefits, serve as an excellent base for reducing the appearance of fine lines and improving overall skin texture. Gels, on the other hand, cater to maintaining skin clarity and preventing acne, which is essential for a youthful complexion. Serums stand out by focusing on specific areas needing intensive care, thereby boosting the skin's natural rejuvenation process.

Athletes and fitness aficionados, who often demand quick-absorbing and non-greasy products, will find gels particularly suitable. The rapid absorption rate ensures that active peptides work efficiently without interfering with physical activities. Serums can provide targeted repair and recovery post-exercise, enhancing skin resilience against environmental stressors such as sun exposure or pollution encountered during outdoor workouts.

Busy professionals, concerned with maintaining mental clarity and coping with cognitive decline, can also benefit from topical peptide products. While the primary focus is often internal health and cognitive enhancers, maintaining a healthy and clear complexion can positively impact self-esteem and mental well-being. Opting for quick and effective skincare, such as gels and serums, integrates seamlessly into a busy routine, providing visible benefits with minimal time investment.

Individuals keen on holistic health will appreciate the natural and scientific blend offered by peptide products. Emphasizing the importance of choosing formulations based on skin type and condition aligns with the holistic perspective of treating the body as an interconnected system. Ensuring that the skincare routine complements overall health practices can enhance both external appearance and internal wellness.

Application Techniques for Topical Products

To effectively apply topical peptide bioregulators, it is essential to understand the techniques that maximize absorption while minimizing waste. Proper usage of these products begins with understanding their chemistry and how they interact with the skin's natural barriers. Peptide bioregulators are designed to penetrate the skin deeply and deliver active ingredients where they are most needed.

One fundamental guideline for maximizing absorption involves applying the product to clean, dry skin. This ensures that no residual oils or dirt block the peptides from entering the skin. It is also beneficial to use a small amount of the product at first, as this helps to gauge how much your skin can absorb without wasting any excess. Applying too much can lead to buildup on the skin's surface, which doesn't enhance the effects but rather leads to unnecessary waste.

Massaging the product into the skin is another effective technique for improving absorption. By gently massaging in circular motions, you not only ensure even distribution but also stimulate blood flow, which can help the peptides reach deeper layers of the skin. Using your fingers or a specialized facial roller enhances this process. Some users find that using upward strokes promotes lifting effects, particularly when targeting areas prone to sagging.

Layering products strategically can significantly enhance the efficacy of topical peptide bioregulators. It's essential to consider the order of application: generally, lighter formulations should be applied before heavier ones. For instance, if you're using a serum followed by a cream, the serum should go on first. This layering allows each product to penetrate effectively without being blocked by thicker substances.

Preparing the skin beforehand is crucial for better product penetration. Exfoliation removes dead skin cells and allows the peptides to access the fresher, more receptive layers underneath. Regular exfoliation, roughly once or twice a week depending on skin sensitivity, keeps the skin in optimal condition to receive active ingredients. Moreover, maintaining a consistent skincare routine that includes cleansing and toning can create an ideal canvas for applying peptide bioregulators.

In addition to preparing the skin, paying attention to its overall moisture levels can enhance peptide absorption. While excessively oily skin might hinder penetration, slightly damp skin can improve the chances of deep absorption. Thus, lightly misting the face with a hydrating toner before applying the peptide product could provide a balance that facilitates better results.

The frequency of applying topical peptide bioregulators is another critical factor. Depending on the desired effects and the specific product formulation, frequency recommendations can vary. Most anti-aging peptides, for example, may be applied once or twice daily—typically in the morning and evening. For performance enhancement or muscle recovery, the application might be more frequent, especially around workout times. However, it's always wise to follow the manufacturer's guidelines and adjust based on personal experience and skin response.

Consistency is key when using peptide bioregulators. It's not just about the immediate effects but the long-term benefits that come from regular application. Documenting your application schedule and any changes in your skin's appearance can help you track effectiveness over time. Keeping a skincare journal can be an invaluable tool for monitoring how your skin responds to different application frequencies and adjusting as needed.

In this chapter, we have explored the various methods of incorporating peptide bioregulators into daily routines. We examined oral supplements like capsules, powders, and liquids, highlighting their unique benefits such as convenience, flexibility in consumption, and fast absorption rates. Additionally, we delved into dosing guidelines, stressing the importance of tailoring dosages to individual health goals and adhering to recommendations for optimal results.

We also discussed the timing of intake and its impact on the efficacy of these supplements, as well as the different forms of topical products available, such as creams, gels, and serums. By understanding the appropriate application techniques, users can maximize the benefits of peptide bioregulators. Overall, this chapter provides a comprehensive guide for health enthusiasts, athletes, busy professionals, and those interested in holistic health approaches to effectively incorporate peptide bioregulators into their wellness practices.

CHAPTER 7

Optimal Dosage and Safety Guidelines

Determining the optimal dosage of peptide bioregulators is critical to maximizing their benefits while ensuring user safety. This chapter delves into the factors influencing effective dosing, emphasizing the importance of individualized regimens. Unlike a one-size-fits-all approach, personalized dosing takes into account various elements such as age, weight, and health conditions. Understanding these aspects allows for more precise control, thereby enhancing the efficacy and safety of peptide use.

In this chapter, we will explore the significance of individual variability in metabolism and how it impacts the effectiveness of peptides. The text will highlight key factors such as genetics, lifestyle, and overall health that influence metabolic rates. Additionally, the chapter provides practical guidelines for creating customized dosage plans, tailored to individual health profiles. By examining clinical research and consulting healthcare professionals, readers will learn how to minimize risks and optimize the outcomes of their peptide regimens.

Determining the Right Dosage

When determining the most effective dosage of peptide bioregulators, understanding individual variability is paramount. Humans differ significantly in their response to various substances due to unique metabolic processes and health statuses. This intrinsic variability means that a one-size-fits-all approach to dosing can often be ineffective or, worse, detrimental. Recognizing individual differences helps ensure that each person receives a dosage tailored to their specific needs, thus maximizing the benefits and minimizing potential risks.

Individual Variability

One of the key aspects of identifying optimal dosages involves acknowledging how personal metabolism plays a role in processing peptides. Metabolism consists of the chemical reactions occurring within our bodies to sustain life, breaking down nutrients to produce energy and build cells. However, the rate at which these reactions occur varies widely from person to person. Factors such as genetics, lifestyle, and overall health can influence metabolic rate. For instance, two individuals with the same weight and height might metabolize nutrients at different rates due to underlying genetic differences. These variations highlight the need for personalized dosing regimens rather than relying solely on standard recommendations.

Different Factors Affecting Metabolism

Age represents a significant factor influencing peptide metabolism. As we age, our metabolic rate declines, affecting how quickly and efficiently our bodies process substances, including peptide bioregulators. Younger individuals typically have faster metabolism compared to older adults, which means they might require different dosages to achieve similar effects. Health enthusiasts interested in anti-aging solutions should especially consider this when determining their peptide intake.

Weight also plays a crucial role in metabolism. Generally, larger individuals may have higher energy requirements and, therefore, might metabolize peptides differently than those with a smaller body mass. It's important for athletes and fitness aficionados looking to enhance performance and muscle growth to take their weight into account when figuring out the ideal dosage. Customized dosage plans based on weight can help in achieving better results while mitigating the risk of over- or under-dosing.

Health conditions further complicate the equation. Chronic illnesses, such as diabetes or thyroid disorders, can impact how the body metabolizes various compounds, including peptides. Individuals with these conditions may require carefully adjusted dosages to avoid adverse effects. Busy professionals concerned about cognitive decline or those seeking to improve mental clarity through peptide use must consider any pre-existing health issues that could alter the effectiveness and safety of their regimen.

Personalized Dosage Regimens

Given the variance in metabolic rates among individuals, personalized dosage regimens are increasingly seen as a superior approach compared to generic recommendations. Personalized doses can offer more precise control over desired outcomes, addressing the individual's specific needs. By tailoring the dosage, users may experience enhanced benefits, such as improved muscle recovery for athletes or greater focus and memory for busy professionals. This customization ensures that the peptide bioregulator's full potential is realized without unnecessary risk.

Creating a personalized dosage regimen involves several steps. Firstly, it is essential to gather comprehensive information about one's health status, lifestyle, and goals. This data serves as the foundation for determining an appropriate starting dose. Next, periodic assessments and adjustments help fine-tune the dosage. Athletes might start with a lower dose and gradually increase it based on their performance and recovery patterns. Similarly, individuals focused on cognitive enhancement might adjust their dosage depending on observed improvements in mental acuity.

Understanding Personal Health Profiles

Having an in-depth understanding of one's health profile is critical when working with peptide bioregulators. This involves knowing medical history, current health conditions, medications being taken, and any potential allergies. A detailed health profile provides valuable insights that guide dosage decisions, ensuring that the interactions between peptides and other factors are thoroughly considered.

For example, someone with a history of cardiovascular issues would need to approach peptide usage cautiously. Certain peptides can affect blood pressure and heart rate, making it essential to tailor the dosage meticulously to avoid exacerbating existing conditions. Likewise, individuals with autoimmune disorders need to consider how peptides might interact with their immune system, balancing efficacy with safety to prevent triggering unwanted immune responses.

By thoroughly understanding their health profiles, users can make informed decisions about peptide dosages. This proactive approach helps in anticipating possible side effects and taking preventive measures to mitigate them. For instance, adjusting doses to align with periodic medical evaluations ensures ongoing safety and efficacy.

In conclusion, the effective dosing of peptide bioregulators demands careful consideration of individual variability. Recognizing the importance of unique metabolic processes, the impact of factors such as age, weight, and health conditions, and the potential benefits of personalized regimens can lead to improved outcomes. Tailoring peptide dosages to fit personal health profiles enhances both the safety and effectiveness of these compounds, making it possible for health enthusiasts, athletes, busy professionals, and those interested in holistic health to optimize their wellness journeys.

Recommended Dosage Guidelines

When considering the appropriate dosage of peptide bioregulators, it's imperative to rely on established thresholds from clinical studies. These thresholds serve as a foundational guide for users and provide a safe starting point for incorporating peptides into their health regimen. Clinical research often provides specific dosages that have been tested for both efficacy and safety across different population groups, including diverse age ranges and health statuses.

For example, clinical trials may indicate that a certain peptide bioregulator is safe and effective at a daily dose of 10 mg in adults. This information is invaluable because it helps to minimize guesswork and ensures that individuals start with a dosage that has been scientifically validated. It's important to recognize that these recommendations are based on controlled environments and specific study parameters. Therefore, applying them in real-world scenarios necessitates a degree of vigilance and adjustment based on personal responses.

Consulting healthcare professionals before embarking on any peptide regimen cannot be overstated. Health experts can offer tailored advice, taking into account individual health profiles, pre-existing conditions, and other medications or supplements currently being used. This personalized guidance is crucial for mitigating risks and enhancing the efficacy of peptide use. For instance, someone with a liver condition might need adjustments in dosing or require more frequent monitoring compared to a healthy individual.

Healthcare providers bring an added layer of expertise by interpreting clinical data in the context of one's unique health status. They can recommend initial dosages, suggest incremental adjustments, and monitor responses, providing a dynamic approach to peptide supplementation. Additionally, they can address any adverse effects that may arise, ensuring timely interventions. By seeking professional advice, users are less likely to experience complications and more likely to achieve their desired health outcomes.

It's also essential to understand that not all peptide bioregulators are created equal. Different peptides may necessitate varying dosages due to their unique properties and mechanisms of action. Some peptides might be potent at lower doses, while others require higher amounts to elicit the desired effect. This variability underscores the importance of adhering to specific guidelines for each type of peptide rather than generalizing dosing recommendations.

For instance, a peptide designed to promote muscle growth might be effective at a different dosage compared to one intended for cognitive enhancement. The variance in dosage requirements highlights the need for precise information and careful planning when integrating multiple peptides into a health routine. This specificity ensures that each peptide is used in a manner that maximizes benefits and minimizes potential risks.

Safeguarding against self-medication is another critical aspect of using peptide bioregulators. While the internet is replete with anecdotal experiences and unverified recommendations, relying on such sources can lead to inappropriate dosing and unintended consequences. Self-medicating without professional supervision can result in either suboptimal efficacy or heightened risk of side effects.

Professional guidance acts as a safeguard against these pitfalls by providing evidence-based dosing instructions and ongoing support. Healthcare professionals can conduct assessments and make necessary adjustments to the dosage, ensuring that the use of peptides remains safe and beneficial. They can also help identify the most suitable peptides based on individual goals and medical history, paving the way for a more informed and judicious approach to peptide use.

Moreover, it's crucial to remain aware of the ongoing advancements in clinical research related to peptide bioregulators. As new studies emerge, dosage recommendations may evolve, reflecting improved understanding and optimized strategies for peptide use. Keeping abreast of these developments through consultation with healthcare professionals ensures that one's regimen remains aligned with the latest scientific insights.

A case in point involves peptides used for anti-aging purposes. Initial studies may have recommended a certain dosage based on early findings. However, subsequent research might reveal a more precise dosage window or uncover additional benefits at different dosages. Staying informed through continuous professional guidance ensures that users can adjust their regimens accordingly and capitalize on the newest findings.

Monitoring and Adjustment

Continuous monitoring and potential dosage adjustments are crucial aspects of using peptide bioregulators effectively and safely. Engaging in periodic evaluations of both their effectiveness and any side effects can significantly enhance health outcomes for users. By systematically assessing how well the peptides are working and identifying any adverse effects, users can fine-tune their regimens to achieve optimal results.

Periodic evaluations allow individuals to understand better how their bodies respond to peptide bioregulators over time. These evaluations should include monitoring physical health markers, mental clarity, and overall well-being. For example, a fitness enthusiast might track muscle recovery rates and performance improvements when taking peptides aimed at enhancing physical capabilities. Concurrently, they should also be aware of any negative reactions such as unusual fatigue or gastrointestinal issues.

The importance of these regular assessments cannot be overstated. Health enthusiasts and athletes alike can benefit from maintaining detailed logs of their experiences and outcomes. This practice can reveal patterns that inform whether adjustments in dosage are necessary. For instance, an individual might find that a lower dose is equally effective and results in fewer side effects. Conversely, some may discover the need for a slight increase to achieve desired benefits. This ongoing process helps mitigate risks associated with long-term use and ensures that the supplements continue to contribute positively to one's health.

Communication with healthcare providers plays an instrumental role in this continuous monitoring process. Regular consultations ensure that users receive professional advice tailored to their unique health needs. Healthcare providers can offer invaluable insights based on medical history, current health status, and specific goals related to peptide use. For example, busy professionals looking to enhance cognitive function can work with their doctors to determine safe dosages that bolster mental clarity without compromising health.

Moreover, healthcare providers can assist in interpreting the data recorded during periodic evaluations. They can identify subtle signs that might indicate the need for dosage adjustments or even temporary discontinuation. Provider-patient communication fosters a collaborative approach, where decisions about peptide use are made based on evidence and expert opinion rather than guesswork. This not only enhances safety but also optimizes the efficacy of the peptides.

Abrupt changes in dosing pose significant risks, which underscores the need for gradual adjustments under professional supervision. Sudden increases or decreases in peptide dosage can lead to unpredictable physiological responses. For example, abruptly stopping a high dose might result in withdrawal-like symptoms, while suddenly increasing the dosage could cause toxicity or exacerbate side effects. Therefore, any dosage modifications should be done gradually and with careful monitoring to ensure the body adapts without adverse effects.

Understanding the potential dangers of abrupt dosage changes is essential for all users. Athletes, for instance, must resist the temptation to quickly scale up doses in pursuit of rapid gains, as this can jeopardize their overall health and athletic performance. Instead, a slow, methodical approach allows the body to acclimate and minimizes the risks of adverse reactions. Professionals, too, need to exercise caution, particularly when using peptides to improve cognitive functions. A sudden shift in dosage could disturb the delicate balance of brain chemistry, leading to unintended consequences.

Accurate documentation of responses and reactions is a cornerstone of successful peptide usage. Keeping a detailed journal that records daily dosages, physical responses, mental state, and any side effects enables users to make informed decisions about their peptide regimen. This practice is especially beneficial for those exploring the anti-aging properties of peptides, as it sheds light on how these compounds affect various aspects of aging over time.

Documenting responses provides a valuable reference that can guide future dosing decisions. Reviewing past entries can help identify trends and correlations that might otherwise go unnoticed. For instance, if a particular dosage consistently corresponds with improved sleep quality or reduced joint pain, that information can be pivotal in crafting a more effective and personalized peptide regimen. Conversely, documenting adverse reactions at certain dosages helps in avoiding those levels in the future, thus preventing unnecessary discomfort or health risks.

Healthcare providers can also utilize these documented logs to adjust treatment plans accurately. With detailed records, providers can pinpoint the exact moments when side effects began or when effectiveness plateaued, making it easier to suggest precise adjustments. This collaborative data-driven approach ensures that both the user and the healthcare provider have a clear understanding of what works best, leading to safer and more effective use of peptide bioregulators.

Common Side Effects

When using peptide bioregulators, it's crucial to be aware of the possible side effects and how to manage them effectively. People who use these substances frequently report several side effects, although not everyone will experience them. This section aims to list common side effects and provide insights into preventive measures for each. Understanding these can help you better manage any adverse symptoms that arise.

One prevalent side effect is headaches. Headaches can range from mild to severe and may occur shortly after administration. To minimize this risk, ensure you are well-hydrated before and after taking peptides. Staying hydrated helps maintain electrolyte balance, which can play a role in preventing headaches. If headaches persist, consider over-the-counter pain relief options, but consult a healthcare provider for advice tailored to your specific health needs.

Injection site reactions are another common concern for users of peptide bioregulators administered through injections. Symptoms can include redness, swelling, or a slight burning sensation at the injection site. These reactions are generally mild and temporary. To prevent such issues, always use a sterile technique for injections. Make sure the injection site is clean, and alternate injection sites regularly to give previously used areas time to heal. Applying a cold compress after the injection can also alleviate pain and reduce swelling.

Gastrointestinal disturbances are also frequently reported. Users may experience symptoms such as nausea, bloating, or diarrhea. These can often be mitigated by adjusting the timing of your dosage or taking the peptide with food if it is safe to do so. Incorporating probiotics into your diet may also help maintain a healthy gut flora, further reducing gastrointestinal discomfort. However, if symptoms persist, consult your healthcare provider to rule out more serious underlying conditions.

While these are some commonly reported side effects, it's important to note that not all users will experience them. Individual variability plays a significant role in how one responds to peptide bioregulators. Factors such as age, overall health, and genetic predispositions can influence the likelihood and severity of side effects. Therefore, just because a side effect is listed doesn't mean it is guaranteed to happen to you.

It's vital for anyone experiencing side effects to report them to their healthcare providers immediately. Timely reporting ensures proper management and reduces the risk of complications. Your healthcare provider can offer guidance on mitigating these effects and may adjust your dosage or recommend alternative peptides if necessary. Open communication with healthcare professionals allows for a more personalized approach to managing side effects and optimizing the benefits of peptide bioregulators.

To further minimize common side effects, certain lifestyle adjustments can be beneficial. A balanced diet rich in essential nutrients supports overall health and can enhance your body's ability to cope with any adverse symptoms. Regular physical activity boosts circulation and promotes more efficient metabolism of peptides, potentially alleviating side effects like headaches and gastrointestinal disturbances. Adequate sleep is another critical factor; it allows your body to recover and repair itself, reducing the likelihood of prolonged adverse reactions.

In addition, consider implementing stress-reduction techniques into your routine. High levels of stress can exacerbate side effects and decrease your overall well-being. Practices such as mindfulness meditation, deep breathing exercises, or yoga can help you maintain a calm and centered mindset. Reducing stress not only improves your emotional health but also has a positive impact on your physical state, making you less susceptible to side effects.

Preventing tolerance buildup is another important aspect to consider when dealing with peptide bioregulators. Over time, your body might become desensitized to the peptide, diminishing its effectiveness. To counter this, it's advisable to cycle your usage. Taking scheduled breaks allows your body to reset, maintaining the efficacy of the peptide. For example, you could use the peptide for a few weeks, followed by a break period before resuming the treatment. Always follow guidelines provided by healthcare professionals regarding cycling to avoid sudden withdrawal effects.

Long-term Safety Considerations

Understanding the long-term safety of peptide supplementation is essential for anyone considering its use, whether they are health enthusiasts, athletes, professionals seeking cognitive enhancement, or individuals interested in holistic health approaches. The current research on the implications of prolonged peptide use offers valuable insights that can help set long-term expectations.

Recent studies have shown varying outcomes depending on the type of peptide and the duration of use. While some peptides demonstrate beneficial effects over extended periods, others may pose risks if not carefully monitored. For instance, growth hormone-releasing peptides (GHRPs) can significantly improve muscle mass and recovery times but may lead to elevated blood pressure or glucose intolerance when used excessively. Similarly, thymus peptides, known for their immune-boosting properties, could potentially alter normal immune responses with long-term use. It's crucial to stay updated with the latest scientific findings to understand these potential impacts comprehensively.

Regular health checkups are paramount when using peptides over an extended period. Consistent medical supervision ensures that any adverse effects are detected early, allowing for timely intervention. This is particularly important because the body's response to peptides can change over time. Health checkups should include comprehensive blood tests, liver function tests, and other diagnostic procedures deemed necessary by a healthcare provider. These assessments help track the body's response to peptide supplementation and adjust dosages as required, ensuring optimal benefits while minimizing risks.

Lifestyle factors play a significant role in mitigating the risks associated with long-term peptide supplementation. A balanced diet, regular exercise, and adequate sleep can enhance the positive effects of peptides and reduce potential side effects. For example, maintaining proper hydration and nutrient levels can support efficient peptide metabolism, preventing issues like dehydration or electrolyte imbalances. Additionally, stress management practices such as meditation or yoga can further bolster the body's resilience, helping mitigate any negative impacts from prolonged peptide use.

Educating oneself on the signs that indicate the need to reassess peptide usage is critical for sustained safety. Users must be aware of any unusual symptoms or changes in their health status that could signify potential issues. Common signs may include persistent fatigue, unexplained weight gain or loss, mood swings, or gastrointestinal disturbances. If any of these symptoms arise, it's essential to consult a healthcare provider promptly. Reassessing peptide usage might involve altering the dosage, switching to a different peptide, or taking a temporary break from supplementation.

Preventive measures are also a crucial aspect of long-term peptide use. Starting with lower dosages allows the body to adapt gradually, minimizing the initial shock to the system. Gradual increases in dosage, under medical supervision, can help identify the optimal level that provides benefits without causing harm. Adherence to established dosage guidelines is vital to prevent overdosing, which can lead to serious health complications. Moreover, maintaining transparency with one's healthcare provider about all supplements and medications being taken can prevent harmful interactions and ensure a holistic approach to health management.

Recognizing and responding to severe reactions promptly is another important guideline. While mild side effects might be manageable, severe reactions require immediate medical attention. Symptoms such as difficulty breathing, severe headaches, chest pain, or extreme swelling at injection sites are red flags that necessitate urgent care. Having an action plan in place, including knowing where the nearest emergency facility is and keeping relevant medical information handy, can make a significant difference in managing such crises effectively.

Determining the right dosage of peptide bioregulators hinges on understanding individual variability and tailoring dosages to fit personal health profiles. This chapter has highlighted key factors such as age, weight, and health conditions that influence how peptides are metabolized. Personalized dosing regimens offer a superior approach compared to generic recommendations, ensuring enhanced benefits with minimized risks. Collecting comprehensive health information and making periodic adjustments allow for fine-tuning the dosage to align with specific goals, whether for muscle recovery, cognitive enhancement, or overall wellness.

Establishing safe starting points from clinical studies and consulting healthcare professionals are fundamental steps in integrating peptides into one's health routine. Individual responses can vary, so ongoing monitoring and adjustment under medical supervision ensure optimal results. Documenting experiences and maintaining open communication with healthcare providers help tailor dosage plans effectively. By considering these guidelines and remaining vigilant about potential side effects, users can harness the full potential of peptide bioregulators safely and effectively, enhancing their overall health and well-being.

CHAPTER 8

Peptide Bioregulators and Immune Function

P eptide bioregulators are instrumental in supporting and enhancing immune health. These small protein-like molecules significantly improve the body's defense mechanisms by stimulating the production of immune cells. This process leads to a more robust immune system that can respond swiftly and effectively to various pathogens and illnesses. By promoting immune cell production, peptide bioregulators play a pivotal role in fortifying the human body against infections and diseases.

This chapter delves into the multifaceted benefits of peptide bioregulators on the immune system, highlighting their capacity to boost immunity and reduce inflammation. It explores how these peptides stimulate the production and function of key immune cells such as T-cells and B-cells. The chapter also examines the scientific evidence supporting the efficacy of peptide bioregulators, discussing their personalized application for different populations, including older adults, athletes, and those with specific health conditions. Additionally, it addresses the holistic health benefits and anti-aging potential of peptide bioregulators, making them an appealing option for individuals looking to enhance overall wellness and longevity.

Enhanced Immune Response

Peptide bioregulators play a crucial role in enhancing the immune system's function. These small protein-like molecules can significantly improve the body's ability to defend itself against various pathogens and illnesses. By stimulating the production of immune cells, peptide bioregulators create a more robust defense mechanism that can respond swiftly and effectively to threats.

One of the most notable benefits of peptide bioregulators is their ability to stimulate the production of immune cells. These cells are essential for identifying and neutralizing harmful invaders like bacteria, viruses, and other pathogens. When the body produces more immune cells, it becomes better equipped to handle infections and diseases. This increased production leads to a stronger, more effective immune response.

A robust immune response is invaluable because it helps the body fend off infections more efficiently. For example, when the immune system is strong, it can quickly recognize and attack harmful microbes before they have a chance to multiply and cause serious illness. This immediate response is crucial in preventing infections from taking hold and spreading throughout the body. Additionally, a strong immune system can help reduce the severity and duration of illnesses, making recovery faster and less complicated.

Increased immune cell production also plays a significant role in helping the body recover from illnesses more quickly. When the body can produce a higher number of immune cells, it can target and eliminate invading pathogens more rapidly. This means that individuals who have a well-supported immune system may experience shorter recovery times from common colds, flu, and other infections. Faster recovery not only improves overall health but also reduces the risk of complications arising from prolonged illness.

Moreover, peptide bioregulators offer the potential for personalized immune support based on individual health needs. Different peptides can be used to target specific areas of the immune system, providing tailored interventions that address unique health challenges. For instance, certain peptides might be more effective at boosting the immune response in older adults, while others could be tailored to support athletes or individuals with specific health conditions. This customization ensures that the immune support provided is as effective and relevant as possible for each person's unique situation.

It is important to understand that the enhancement of immune function through peptide bioregulators is supported by scientific evidence. Research has shown that these molecules can influence various aspects of the immune system, including the activation and proliferation of key immune cells like T-cells and B-cells. Such studies highlight the potential of peptides to serve as powerful tools in maintaining and improving immune health across different populations.

For health enthusiasts and individuals interested in anti-aging solutions, peptide bioregulators present an appealing option for enhancing overall wellness and longevity. By supporting immune function, these peptides can help protect against age-related decline in immune health. This protection is vital for maintaining resilience against infections and diseases that become more prevalent as we age.

Athletes and fitness aficionados can also benefit from the immune-boosting properties of peptide bioregulators. A strong immune system is crucial for maintaining peak performance, muscle growth, and recovery times. Athletes often push their bodies to the limit, which can sometimes weaken the immune system and make them more susceptible to infections. By incorporating peptide bioregulators into their regimen, they can enhance their immune defenses and minimize downtime due to illness.

Busy professionals concerned about cognitive decline can find value in peptide bioregulators as well. A healthy immune system is closely linked to cognitive function since chronic inflammation and immune dysregulation can negatively impact mental clarity and memory. By supporting immune health, peptide bioregulators may contribute to better focus and cognitive performance, helping professionals maintain productivity and mental sharpness.

Furthermore, individuals interested in holistic health approaches will appreciate the natural and targeted benefits that peptide bioregulators offer. Unlike conventional medicines that might have broad and non-specific effects, peptides can provide specific and effective support to the immune system without the side effects associated with some pharmaceutical interventions. This makes peptide bioregulators a desirable option for those seeking alternative and complementary methods to enhance their health and well-being.

Regulation of Cytokines

In the intricate dance of immune function, peptides play a pivotal role by influencing the balance of cytokines, which are crucial in signaling immune responses. To understand this dynamic, it's essential first to grasp what cytokines are and why they matter. Cytokines are small proteins released by cells that have a specific impact on the interactions and communications between cells.

They act as messengers that facilitate the immune system's response to infections, inflammation, trauma, and other stimuli.

One key aspect of maintaining proper health is regulating cytokine levels. When cytokine levels are balanced, the immune system can effectively respond to threats without overreacting. Overactive cytokine responses can lead to conditions like allergies and autoimmune diseases, where the body attacks its own tissues. Peptides help modulate these responses, ensuring that cytokine levels stay within an optimal range, thus preventing such detrimental overreactions. This modulation is particularly significant for individuals prone to allergic reactions, as properly balanced cytokines mean fewer and less severe allergic responses.

Moreover, proper cytokine regulation is vital for enhancing the body's adaptive immune responses. The adaptive immune system is responsible for targeting specific pathogens with high precision, thanks to the memory of past encounters. Peptides influence cytokine production, promoting a more effective and tailored immune response. For instance, when the body recognizes a pathogen it has encountered before, peptides help modulate cytokine release to signal for a swift and targeted attack. This precise response allows for more efficient pathogen elimination and quicker recovery.

Maintaining a balance in cytokine levels is not just about immediate immune responses; it's crucial for long-term health and immune efficiency. Chronic imbalance in cytokine levels can lead to prolonged inflammation and other health issues. Inflammation is a natural part of the immune response, but when it becomes chronic, it can contribute to various diseases, including cardiovascular disease, diabetes, and even cancer. By helping maintain cytokine balance, peptides play a role in reducing the risk of these chronic conditions, supporting overall longevity and wellness.

Understanding how cytokines function and how their balance can be maintained through peptide regulation opens the door to new therapeutic strategies for managing immune disorders. Many modern therapies for immune-related conditions, such as rheumatoid arthritis and multiple sclerosis, focus on modulating cytokine activity. Peptides offer a promising avenue in this regard, providing a natural means to adjust cytokine levels and improve outcomes for individuals with such disorders. Therapies that harness the power of peptides could potentially offer more targeted and fewer side-effect-prone treatments compared to traditional pharmaceuticals.

To elaborate further, consider how peptides interact with different types of cytokines. There are pro-inflammatory cytokines, which promote inflammation, and anti-inflammatory cytokines, which suppress it. A healthy immune system maintains a delicate balance between these two types. If pro-inflammatory cytokines dominate, the result is excessive inflammation, which, if persistent, can damage tissues and organs. On the other hand, if anti-inflammatory cytokines are too prevalent, the immune system might become underactive, failing to respond adequately to genuine threats. Peptides can help fine-tune this balance, ensuring that the immune system remains active enough to protect against pathogens but not so active that it causes harm.

Research has shown that certain peptides can selectively increase or decrease the production of specific cytokines. For example, thymosin alpha-1 is a peptide known to enhance the production of various cytokines involved in stimulating immune responses. This peptide has been studied for its potential to boost immune function in individuals with compromised immunity, such as those undergoing chemotherapy or those with chronic viral infections. By increasing the levels of beneficial cytokines, thymosin alpha-1 helps strengthen the body's defenses, illustrating the practical application of cytokine modulation through peptides.

Additionally, peptides can assist in creating a more adaptable and resilient immune system. This adaptability is critical for athletes and fitness enthusiasts who continuously push their bodies to the limit. During intense physical activity, the body experiences temporary spikes in pro-inflammatory cytokines as part of the repair process. However, uncontrolled inflammation can lead to prolonged recovery times and increased injury risk. Peptides can help manage this inflammatory response, promoting faster recovery and better performance. By modulating cytokine levels, peptides ensure that the immune system supports muscle repair and growth without causing excessive inflammation.

For busy professionals and individuals concerned about cognitive decline, maintaining optimal cytokine levels through peptide regulation can also support brain health. Neuroinflammation, often driven by imbalanced cytokine levels, is associated with cognitive impairment and neurodegenerative diseases like Alzheimer's. By promoting a balanced cytokine environment, peptides may help prevent or mitigate such conditions, contributing to improved mental clarity, focus, and overall cognitive function.

Promoting Natural Killer Cell Activity

The enhancement of natural killer (NK) cell activity by peptide bioregulators represents a significant advancement in our understanding of immune function. NK cells are crucial components of the innate immune system, known for their ability to target and destroy virally infected cells and cancerous tumors. By boosting NK cell activity, peptide bioregulators can significantly enhance the body's capacity to fight off these threats.

To appreciate the importance of NK cells, it's essential to understand their role in immunity. NK cells act as the body's first line of defense against infections and malignancies. They possess the unique ability to recognize stressed cells in the absence of antibodies and MHC, allowing for a faster immune response compared to other immune cells. This rapid response is particularly vital in eliminating virally infected cells before they can replicate and spread, as well as in targeting tumor cells that may arise spontaneously.

Increased NK cell activity translates into a more robust elimination of virally infected cells and tumors. Peptide bioregulators facilitate this process by enhancing the cytotoxic capabilities of NK cells, improving their ability to identify and destroy harmful cells. Several studies have demonstrated that specific peptides can upregulate the expression of activating receptors on NK cells, such as NKG2D, which play a pivotal role in recognizing and binding to targets. This upregulation results in heightened cytolytic activity, thereby enhancing the overall immune surveillance and response.

Moreover, enhanced NK cell function can provide a faster and more effective immune response to various threats. The swift action of NK cells is critical in controlling early stages of infection and inhibiting tumor growth, providing time for the adaptive immune system to mount a more specific response. Peptides that enhance NK cell functions can thus be seen as catalysts, speeding up the immune response and ensuring that threats are neutralized promptly. This faster response not only limits the spread of infections but also reduces the likelihood of secondary complications arising from prolonged immune battles.

Understanding the dynamics of NK cell activity is also instrumental in developing targeted therapies for immunocompromised individuals. For those with weakened immune systems, such as patients undergoing chemotherapy or those with chronic illnesses, enhancing NK cell function could offer a lifeline. By leveraging peptide bioregulators, it is possible to selectively bolster the innate immune response, providing these patients with a better chance of fighting off infections and preventing disease progression. Research into the specific mechanisms through which peptides influence NK cells can guide the creation of personalized treatments tailored to individual needs.

Another critical aspect of increasing NK cell activity is its impact on overall immune vigilance and health. A heightened state of immune readiness means the body is constantly prepared to fend off new and recurring threats. This continuous vigilance is particularly important in an era where new pathogens emerge regularly, as seen with recent global health crises. By promoting robust NK cell activity, peptide bioregulators ensure that the immune system remains agile and responsive, capable of adapting to various challenges swiftly.

Furthermore, the role of peptides in modulating NK cell function extends beyond immediate immune responses. Long-term enhancement of NK cell activity can contribute to sustained immune health, reducing the incidence of chronic diseases linked to immune dysfunction. Conditions such as autoimmune disorders, chronic viral infections, and even certain cancers can be mitigated through improved NK cell function. Thus, the use of peptide bioregulators not only addresses acute immune challenges but also provides long-term benefits for overall health.

Additionally, athletes and fitness enthusiasts can benefit from enhanced NK cell activity. Physical exertion and stress can temporarily suppress immune function, making individuals more susceptible to infections. By incorporating peptide bioregulators that target NK cells, athletes can maintain a strong immune defense, promoting quicker recovery times and sustained performance levels. This application underscores the versatility of peptide bioregulators in enhancing health across different populations, from those seeking longevity and wellness to high-performance individuals aiming for optimal physical condition.

Support for Mucosal Immunity

Peptide bioregulators play a crucial role in strengthening mucosal surfaces, which serve as key barriers against pathogens. Mucosal immunity encompasses the immune functions associated with mucosal surfaces such as those lining the gastrointestinal tract, respiratory system, and other body cavities. By enhancing these surfaces' integrity, peptides contribute significantly to an individual's overall health.

Firstly, stronger mucosal immunity is instrumental in reducing the incidence of gastrointestinal and respiratory infections. The mucosal surfaces act as the body's first line of defense, preventing pathogens from invading deeper tissues. Peptides bolster this defense by improving the structural integrity and functional capabilities of the mucosal cells. For example, specific peptides can enhance the production of mucus, which traps pathogens and facilitates their removal from the body. Additionally, peptides stimulate the production of immunoglobulins, particularly IgA, which neutralize harmful microorganisms in the mucosal layers. The outcome is fewer instances of common infections such as colds, flu, and gastroenteritis, thanks to the fortified mucosal barrier.

Enhancing intestinal barrier functions also plays a critical role in overall immune health. The intestinal barrier is composed of tightly joined epithelial cells that prevent harmful substances from entering the bloodstream while allowing nutrient absorption. Peptides strengthen these barriers by promoting cell regeneration and repair processes. When the intestinal barrier is compromised, it can lead to conditions like leaky gut syndrome, where toxins and bacteria penetrate the bloodstream, triggering systemic inflammation and weakening the immune response. By maintaining the integrity of the intestinal mucosa, peptides help prevent these issues, thereby supporting a healthier immune system.

Supporting mucosal immunity has further benefits in maintaining a balanced microbiome. The human microbiome, particularly within the gut, consists of a diverse community of beneficial microbes that play significant roles in digestion, vitamin production, and immune function. Peptides influence the composition and activity of these microbial populations. They can inhibit the growth of pathogenic bacteria while promoting the proliferation of beneficial bacteria, creating a balanced and healthy gut microbiome. This balance is essential because a disrupted microbiome can lead to dysbiosis, which is associated with various health problems including inflammatory bowel disease, obesity, and even mental health disorders. Thus, peptides indirectly support immune function by ensuring a stable and thriving microbiome.

Robust mucosal defenses also contribute to long-term protection against environmental pathogens. In our daily lives, we are constantly exposed to potential threats from pollutants, allergens, and infectious agents. Mucosal surfaces act as gatekeepers that filter out these harmful substances before they can cause harm. Peptides enhance the resilience of these surfaces through several mechanisms. They can induce the expression of antimicrobial peptides (AMPs) naturally produced by the body. These AMPs exhibit broad-spectrum activity against bacteria, viruses, and fungi, providing a powerful layer of defense. Additionally, certain peptides have anti-inflammatory properties that help modulate the mucosal immune response, preventing excessive inflammation that can damage tissues and impair defense mechanisms.

The strengthening of mucosal surfaces through peptides not only boosts immediate immune defense but also offers lasting health benefits. By continuously supporting mucosal immunity, peptides contribute to a more resilient and adaptable immune system capable of quickly responding to new threats. This is especially important for individuals who are frequently exposed to high-risk environments, such as athletes, busy professionals, and those seeking holistic health approaches.

Moreover, peptide bioregulators can be tailored to address specific needs, allowing for personalized interventions that optimize mucosal immunity based on individual health profiles. This adaptability makes peptides a versatile tool in the pursuit of enhanced immune function and overall well-being.

Anti-Inflammatory Properties

Peptide bioregulators play a crucial role in mitigating inflammation, contributing significantly to overall health and wellness. These small protein fragments regulate various biological processes, including the body's inflammatory response. Many peptides exhibit properties that help reduce chronic inflammation, a condition linked to numerous diseases such as cardiovascular disorders, diabetes, and autoimmune conditions.

Chronic inflammation is a state of persistent, low-level inflammation that can go unnoticed for years, silently damaging tissues and organs. Peptides like thymosin beta-4, BPC-157, and LL-37 are known for their anti-inflammatory effects. Thymosin beta-4, for instance, has been shown to minimize inflammation by reducing levels of pro-inflammatory cytokines, proteins that promote inflammation. Similarly, BPC-157, derived from stomach enzymes, promotes healing and reduces inflammation in gut tissues, making it beneficial for individuals with inflammatory bowel disease. LL-37, an antimicrobial peptide, not only fights infections but also modulates inflammation, enhancing tissue repair and immune regulation.

Reducing chronic inflammation is vital for preventing numerous diseases, including autoimmune disorders. Autoimmune diseases occur when the immune system mistakenly attacks healthy cells, mistaking them for harmful pathogens. Conditions like rheumatoid arthritis, lupus, and multiple sclerosis are examples of autoimmune disorders characterized by chronic inflammation. By reducing inflammation, peptides help modulate the immune system's activity, preventing it from becoming overactive and attacking the body's own tissues. This modulation is essential in maintaining a balanced immune response, thereby reducing the risk of developing autoimmune diseases.

Lower inflammation levels also improve recovery and enhance physical performance, which is particularly relevant for athletes and fitness enthusiasts. Inflammation is a natural response to muscle damage caused by intense workouts. However, excessive inflammation can lead to prolonged soreness and delayed recovery. Peptides such as IGF-1 (Insulin-like Growth Factor 1) and collagen peptides can aid in muscle repair and reduce inflammation. IGF-1 promotes muscle growth and repair by stimulating protein synthesis and decreasing inflammatory markers. Collagen peptides support joint and connective tissue health, reducing inflammation and pain, thus enhancing overall physical performance and recovery times.

Effective inflammation management through peptide bioregulators results in a well-regulated immune response against pathogens while minimizing tissue damage. The immune system is designed to protect the body from infections and injuries by initiating an inflammatory response. However, unchecked inflammation can cause more harm than good, leading to tissue damage and impaired function. Peptides help balance this inflammatory response, ensuring that it remains effective without becoming destructive. For example, the peptide thymosin alpha-1 boosts immune cell activity while simultaneously controlling inflammation, providing a dual benefit of enhanced immunity and reduced inflammation.

In addition to these specific peptides, lifestyle factors such as diet, exercise, and stress management can influence inflammation levels. Incorporating anti-inflammatory foods like fatty fish, leafy greens, and berries into one's diet can complement the benefits of peptide bioregulators. Regular physical activity and adequate sleep also play significant roles in managing inflammation. Stress reduction techniques such as meditation, yoga, and deep breathing can further aid in reducing chronic inflammation.

Furthermore, ongoing research continues to uncover new peptides with potential anti-inflammatory properties. Scientists are exploring peptides derived from various sources, including plants, marine organisms, and synthetic analogs, to develop novel treatments for inflammation-related conditions. This expanding knowledge base offers hope for more targeted and effective interventions in the future.

In this chapter, we delved into the significant role peptide bioregulators play in supporting and enhancing immune health. We examined how these small protein-like molecules boost the production of immune cells, leading to a stronger immune response capable of swiftly identifying and neutralizing pathogens. Additionally, we looked at the ability of peptides to personalize immune support, tailoring their effects to meet individual health needs and addressing specific challenges.

Furthermore, we explored the anti-inflammatory properties of peptide bioregulators and their impact on reducing chronic inflammation. By balancing cytokine levels, peptides help prevent overactive immune responses that can lead to allergies or autoimmune diseases. This modulation supports long-term immune efficiency and overall wellness. Whether for health enthusiasts, athletes, busy professionals, or individuals seeking holistic health approaches, peptide bioregulators offer promising tools for enhancing immunity and improving quality of life.

CHAPTER 9

Peptide Bioregulators for Cardiovascular Health

Peptide bioregulators are potent agents that hold significant potential for improving cardiovascular health. These peptides, which are short chains of amino acids, have garnered attention for their unique ability to influence various functions within the cardiovascular system, making them a subject of interest among health enthusiasts, athletes, and professionals alike.

In this chapter, we will explore how peptide bioregulators enhance blood circulation, contributing to heart health and vascular function. The discussion will cover their role in promoting nitric oxide synthesis, which helps in vasodilation and ensures efficient blood flow throughout the body. We will also examine the implications of improved blood circulation on overall tissue health, cardiovascular endurance, and blood pressure regulation. Additionally, the chapter will highlight the benefits of peptides in preventing atherosclerosis, supporting other bodily systems, and aligning with holistic health approaches. By delving into scientific research and practical examples, this chapter aims to provide a comprehensive understanding of the benefits and applications of peptide bioregulators for maintaining cardiovascular wellness.

Improving Blood Circulation

Peptide bioregulators have emerged as potent agents in enhancing blood flow and circulation, thus significantly contributing to cardiovascular health. At the heart of their functionality is their ability to promote the synthesis of nitric oxide (NO). Nitric oxide plays an essential role in cardiovascular health by acting as a vasodilator. This means it helps relax and widen blood vessels, making it easier for blood to flow through them. By promoting NO synthesis, peptide bioregulators help ensure that blood vessels remain flexible and healthy.

When blood vessels are dilated, it allows for increased blood flow. This enhanced circulation ensures that oxygen and vital nutrients are delivered more efficiently to tissues throughout the body. Improved nutrient delivery is crucial because it supports cellular functions and fosters overall tissue health. In essence, peptide bioregulators contribute to maintaining an optimal internal environment where cells can thrive and perform their duties effectively.

One significant benefit of improved blood flow is its impact on cardiovascular endurance during physical activity. Athletes and fitness enthusiasts often seek ways to enhance their performance and stamina. When blood flows freely, muscles receive a continuous supply of oxygen and nutrients, which is particularly important during prolonged or intense exercise. Enhanced circulation means that muscles can work harder and longer without tiring quickly, thereby boosting athletic performance and endurance.

Additionally, enhanced blood flow brought about by peptide bioregulators has another critical advantage—it can help reduce blood pressure. Blood pressure is the force exerted by circulating blood against the walls of the body's arteries, and high blood pressure is a known risk factor for many cardiovascular diseases. By promoting vasodilation, peptide bioregulators help lower this force, easing the heart's workload and reducing the risk of conditions such as hypertension. Hypertension, if left unmanaged, can lead to severe complications like stroke or heart attack. Hence, maintaining a normal blood pressure level is fundamental to cardiovascular health.

Increased nitric oxide production not only aids in lowering blood pressure but also plays a key role in overall vascular health. Healthy blood vessels are less likely to develop atherosclerosis, a condition characterized by the hardening and narrowing of the arteries due to plaque buildup. Peptide bioregulators, by boosting NO levels, help keep arteries clear and elastic, thus preventing conditions that can impede blood flow and elevate the risk of cardiovascular incidents.

The benefits of peptide bioregulators extend beyond just vascular health. By ensuring efficient blood flow and nutrient delivery, they indirectly support other bodily systems as well. For instance, proper circulation is vital for cognitive function. The brain requires a consistent supply of oxygen and nutrients to operate at peak efficiency. Enhanced circulation ensures that these needs are met, potentially improving focus, memory, and mental clarity. This can be particularly beneficial for busy professionals who require sustained cognitive performance and alertness throughout the day.

Furthermore, the role of peptide bioregulators in promoting cardiovascular health aligns with holistic health approaches. These peptides offer a natural and non-invasive way to improve heart health, making them attractive to individuals interested in alternative medicine and wellness supplements. As natural substances, they tend to have fewer side effects compared to traditional pharmaceutical interventions, making them a safer option for long-term use.

Given the demanding lifestyles many lead today, managing stress and its impact on cardiovascular health is paramount. Stress can trigger a cascade of physiological responses that increase heart rate and blood pressure. By promoting relaxation and reducing the physiological impacts of stress, peptide bioregulators can indirectly support heart health. The vasodilating effect of nitric oxide helps counteract the constricting effects of stress hormones on blood vessels, thereby helping to maintain normal blood pressure levels even in stressful situations.

Moreover, the potential of peptide bioregulators in supporting cardiovascular health is backed by emerging scientific research. Studies have shown that peptides can play a role in modulating various biological pathways, including those involved in vascular health. Researchers continue to investigate how these compounds can be optimized and utilized for maximum benefit, paving the way for innovative treatments and preventive measures for cardiovascular diseases.

Ultimately, the integration of peptide bioregulators into one's health regimen should be approached with consideration and guidance from healthcare professionals. While the benefits highlighted here are promising, individual responses to these peptides can vary. Personalized medical advice ensures that one can harness the advantages of peptide bioregulators safely and effectively.

Elevating Heart Efficiency

Optimizing cardiac output through the use of peptide bioregulators is a fascinating aspect of cardiovascular health that holds immense promise. Peptides, which are short chains of amino acids, have been shown to play crucial roles in various bodily functions, including heart efficiency. By optimizing cardiac output, peptides make the heart more efficient at pumping blood, leading to numerous benefits.

When the heart becomes more efficient, it requires less energy to perform its function. This reduction in energy expenditure decreases the overall workload and strain on the heart. In simpler terms, an efficiently functioning heart doesn't have to work as hard to pump blood throughout the body. This can be particularly beneficial for older adults or those with preexisting heart conditions, where minimizing cardiac strain is crucial for maintaining optimal health. A heart that operates efficiently is akin to a well-oiled machine, performing its tasks without unnecessary wear and tear. This means the organ remains healthier for longer periods, reducing the likelihood of potential damage or failure over time.

Another critical benefit of increased cardiac efficiency is the enhancement of stamina during physical exertion. When the heart pumps blood more effectively, oxygen and nutrients are more readily delivered to muscles and other tissues. This improved delivery system allows individuals to enjoy higher levels of endurance and stamina. Athletes and fitness enthusiasts may particularly appreciate this advantage, as it can lead to improved performance and faster recovery times after workouts. For instance, consider a marathon runner who relies heavily on cardiovascular endurance. With a more efficient heart, the runner can maintain a steady pace for more extended periods, potentially achieving better race times and overall performance.

Enhanced heart function also plays a significant role in decreasing the risk of heart-related complications. Conditions such as heart attacks, strokes, and heart failure often stem from the heart's inability to function correctly. By using peptide bioregulators to optimize cardiac performance, individuals can significantly lower their risk of developing these severe health issues. Additionally, a healthy heart is better equipped to handle stressors, whether they come from physical activity or everyday life challenges. The reduced strain on the heart minimizes the likelihood of acute stress responses that could otherwise trigger adverse cardiac events.

Moreover, optimizing cardiac performance contributes substantially to long-term cardiovascular health. Over time, the cumulative effects of a more efficient heart translate into a robust cardiovascular system less prone to disease and dysfunction. Maintaining heart health is essential not only for longevity but also for quality of life. Individuals who invest in their cardiac health through methods such as peptide bioregulation tend to experience lower incidences of chronic illnesses like hypertension and atherosclerosis. They also enjoy more active lifestyles, as a healthy heart supports a wider range of physical activities.

One practical example of how peptides can aid in cardiac efficiency is their potential role in improving mitochondrial function within heart cells. Mitochondria, known as the powerhouses of the cell, are responsible for producing the energy required for cellular functions. Peptides can enhance mitochondrial efficiency, ensuring that heart cells generate adequate energy with minimal waste. This biochemical optimization directly translates into a heart that performs its duties more effectively, reinforcing the previously mentioned benefits.

Furthermore, peptides may also help regulate the balance of electrolytes within heart cells. Electrolytes like potassium, calcium, and sodium are vital for maintaining the electrical charges necessary for proper heartbeats. An imbalance in these electrolytes can lead to arrhythmias or irregular heartbeats. By regulating these elements, peptides ensure a consistent and stable heartbeat, further enhancing the overall efficiency of the cardiovascular system.

In addition to their direct impact on heart cells, peptides can positively influence the vascular system. Efficient cardiac output isn't just about the heart itself; it's also about the network of arteries and veins that distribute blood throughout the body. Some peptides can promote vasodilation, or the widening of blood vessels, which reduces resistance against the heart's pumping action. This makes it easier for the heart to circulate blood, thereby enhancing its efficiency. A well-functioning vascular system ensures that all organs receive an adequate supply of oxygenated blood, contributing to their optimal function and overall health.

Peptides may also support the production of essential proteins and enzymes involved in heart function. For example, certain peptides can stimulate the synthesis of collagen, a structural protein that helps maintain the integrity and flexibility of blood vessels. Strong, flexible blood vessels are less likely to suffer from blockages or ruptures, both of which can lead to cardiovascular complications. By supporting the structural components of the heart and circulatory system, peptides help ensure long-term robustness and resilience.

Given these multifaceted benefits, it's clear that incorporating peptides into one's health regimen offers significant advantages for cardiovascular health. Whether you're a health enthusiast looking to improve your overall wellness, an athlete aiming for peak performance, or a busy professional concerned about long-term heart health, peptides provide a scientifically-backed method to enhance cardiac efficiency. While ongoing research continues to unravel the full potential of these compounds, current evidence strongly supports their role in promoting a healthy, efficient heart.

Influencing Endothelial Function

Peptide bioregulators, small chains of amino acids, have garnered attention for their potential to bolster cardiovascular health through their effects on the endothelium. The endothelium is the inner lining of blood vessels and plays a crucial role in maintaining vascular health. This section delves into the positive impacts peptide bioregulators can have on endothelial function, highlighting how this can lead to reduced plaque formation, improved vascular responsiveness, and overall circulatory system integrity.

Firstly, enhanced endothelial function is linked to reduced plaque formation and atherosclerosis. Plaque buildup within arteries can narrow and harden them, leading to atherosclerosis, a key contributor to heart attacks and strokes. Peptide bioregulators aid in maintaining the health and functionality of the endothelium by promoting cellular repair and regeneration. This helps prevent the adhesion of inflammatory cells and lipids to the endothelial walls, reducing the risk of plaque formation. Consequently, keeping the endothelium in good condition can stave off the development of atherosclerosis, thereby supporting overall cardiovascular health.

Improved endothelial health also contributes to better vascular responsiveness. The endothelium produces nitric oxide, a molecule essential for vasodilation – the widening of blood vessels. Vasodilation is necessary for regulating blood pressure and ensuring that organs and tissues receive adequate oxygen and nutrients. Peptide bioregulators enhance the production and release of nitric oxide, thereby improving the ability of blood vessels to dilate efficiently. This leads to better regulation of blood pressure and improves the body's response to physical stressors such as exercise or other demanding activities. For athletes and fitness enthusiasts, this translates to enhanced performance and endurance due to optimal blood flow and nutrient delivery during workouts.

Vigilant endothelial function supports overall circulatory system integrity and heart health. A well-functioning endothelium ensures that the blood flows smoothly without unnecessary friction or turbulence, which could otherwise lead to damage or clot formation. Healthy endothelial cells produce anticoagulant factors that prevent unwanted clots, contributing to a balanced hemostatic environment. Peptide bioregulators help maintain this balance, supporting the integrity and resilience of the vascular system. By doing so, they reduce the risk of complications such as thrombosis and embolisms, which can be life-threatening if not managed properly.

Furthermore, the maintenance of a healthy blood vessel lining is critical for heart health. The endothelium acts as a barrier between the blood and the rest of the vessel wall, controlling the exchange of substances and protecting against harmful elements. Peptide bioregulators aid in preserving this protective layer, ensuring that it remains intact and functional. This is particularly important in preventing the onset of conditions that can compromise cardiovascular health, such as hypertension and chronic inflammation. By promoting the health of the endothelial lining, peptide bioregulators contribute significantly to the longevity and robustness of the heart and vascular system.

Thromboresistance

Maintaining healthy blood viscosity and preventing unwanted clot formation are critical in safeguarding cardiovascular health. Peptide bioregulators have shown promise in supporting these vital functions, offering multiple benefits for those seeking to enhance their overall well-being.

Firstly, reducing the risk of clot formation is crucial in lowering the incidences of heart attacks and strokes. Blood clots can obstruct blood flow to the heart or brain, leading to these potentially life-threatening conditions. By ensuring that blood remains fluid and less prone to clotting, peptide bioregulators help maintain an unobstructed vascular system. This not only decreases the likelihood of acute events but also contributes to long-term cardiovascular health. Individuals who manage to keep their blood free-flowing face a diminished threat of sudden blockages that could lead to severe health crises.

The consistent and vigilant flow of blood through the arteries and veins is another cornerstone of overall cardiovascular function. It ensures that oxygen and essential nutrients are delivered efficiently to tissues throughout the body. Peptide bioregulators can support this process by modulating various mechanisms responsible for maintaining optimal blood flow. A steady and smooth circulation system enhances endurance and general physical performance. For athletes and fitness enthusiasts, this translates into improved stamina and quicker recovery times after strenuous activities.

Moreover, promoting a more fluid blood environment assists significantly in the recovery from vascular injuries. When blood maintains an appropriate level of viscosity, it can better navigate through damaged or healing vessels without causing further complications. Vascular injuries can often lead to inflammation and swelling, which may impede proper circulation. Peptide bioregulators help mitigate these effects by fostering a blood environment conducive to healing. This is especially beneficial for individuals recovering from surgeries or those with chronic conditions that affect vascular integrity. By enhancing blood flow, these peptides facilitate the repair processes, thus speeding up recovery and restoring normal function more swiftly.

Peptide bioregulators also play an essential role in the ongoing maintenance of thromboresistance within the bloodstream. Thromboresistance refers to the ability of blood to resist clot formation under normal physiological conditions. Maintaining this resistance is crucial for preventing unwanted clots that could disrupt the cardiovascular system. Peptide bioregulators contribute by interacting with various proteins and cells involved in the clotting cascade, ensuring that the blood remains balanced and less likely to coagulate inappropriately. This balance is a key factor in preserving cardiovascular health over the long term, particularly for those at higher risk of clot-related issues.

Additionally, these peptides have multifaceted effects on blood quality and composition. They often exert anti-inflammatory properties, helping to minimize chronic inflammation that can exacerbate clotting risks. Inflammation within the blood vessels can create an environment more conducive to clot formation, so reducing this inflammation is a critical step in maintaining a healthy circulatory system. The holistic approach of peptide bioregulators addresses not just one aspect but several interconnected factors that influence cardiovascular health. This comprehensive action makes them valuable allies in the pursuit of heart health and longevity.

For the health-conscious individual aiming to implement evidence-based strategies to enhance cardiovascular wellness, incorporating peptide bioregulators can be a prudent choice. Their ability to reduce clot formation, support continuous and effective blood flow, aid in recovery from vascular injuries, and maintain thromboresistance underscores their potential as powerful tools in cardiovascular care. These benefits are particularly relevant for those who might be at an elevated risk of heart attacks and strokes, such as older adults, individuals with a family history of cardiovascular disease, and those living with conditions like diabetes or hypertension.

Reducing the Risk of Cardiovascular Diseases

Peptide bioregulators are emerging as a powerful tool in the fight against cardiovascular disease, thanks to their ability to support heart health through several mechanisms. By positively influencing lipid profiles, they help manage cholesterol levels and prevent conditions like atherosclerosis. This is particularly significant because balanced lipid levels can lower the risks associated with clogged arteries, potentially leading to heart attacks and strokes.

The role of peptides in cholesterol regulation cannot be understated. High levels of low-density lipoprotein (LDL) cholesterol contribute to the buildup of plaques in arterial walls—a condition known as atherosclerosis. Peptides can assist in maintaining healthy cholesterol levels by enhancing the body's natural lipid metabolism, promoting the reduction of LDL cholesterol while supporting higher levels of high-density lipoprotein (HDL) cholesterol. This balance is crucial in preventing the formation of arterial plaques that can restrict blood flow and increase the risk of cardiovascular events. Incorporating peptide bioregulators into one's health regimen could serve as a proactive measure for maintaining a healthy cardiovascular system.

Another vital aspect of peptide bioregulators is their anti-inflammatory properties. Chronic inflammation plays a critical role in the development of various cardiovascular diseases. Inflammation can damage the endothelium, the inner lining of blood vessels, making them more susceptible to plaque formation and clotting. Peptides help combat this issue by reducing inflammatory markers in the body and protecting the vascular system from chronic inflammation. This protective effect is not only beneficial for immediate heart health but also aids in maintaining long-term cardiovascular vitality.

Inflammation within the cardiovascular system can lead to a weakened heart muscle and damaged blood vessels, which compromises overall heart function. By mitigating these inflammatory processes, peptides help safeguard the heart and blood vessels from enduring damage. This helps ensure that blood vessels remain flexible and resilient, capable of efficiently managing blood pressure and sustaining healthy circulation.

Additionally, peptides play a significant role in optimizing metabolic health, which is another cornerstone of cardiovascular wellness. Poor metabolic health, often characterized by obesity and type 2 diabetes, places a heavy burden on the heart. These conditions are associated with increased blood pressure, elevated cholesterol levels, and excessive strain on the cardiovascular system. Peptide bioregulators enhance metabolism by improving glucose utilization and energy production, which assists in weight management and reduces the risk of metabolic syndrome—an array of conditions that elevate the risk of heart disease.

A well-regulated metabolism not only keeps body weight in check but also ensures that the body's organs, including the heart, receive an adequate supply of nutrients and oxygen. Efficient metabolic processes mean less fat storage and a reduced likelihood of developing obesity-related complications that stress the cardiovascular system. Individuals who are able to maintain a healthy metabolism through the use of peptides will find themselves better positioned to avoid the cumulative effects of metabolic disorders on heart health.

Stress management is another area where peptide bioregulators show promise. Chronic stress is a well-known risk factor for hypertension and cardiovascular disease. Under stress, the body releases cortisol and other stress hormones that can raise blood pressure and heart rate. Over time, this heightened state of alertness can take a toll on the cardiovascular system. Peptides help modulate the body's stress response, leading to lower levels of cortisol and other stress-related chemicals. This results in a more relaxed state, which positively influences heart health by lowering blood pressure and decreasing the risk of stress-induced cardiac events.

By helping to manage stress more effectively, peptides encourage healthier lifestyle choices. Lower stress levels generally correspond to improved sleep patterns, better dietary habits, and greater inclination towards physical activity—all of which have beneficial effects on cardiovascular health. Less stress means less wear and tear on the heart and a decreased likelihood of developing stress-related cardiovascular issues.

This chapter has illustrated the significant benefits of peptide bioregulators for heart health and vascular function. By promoting nitric oxide synthesis, these peptides aid in relaxing and widening blood vessels, thereby improving blood circulation and lowering blood pressure. Enhanced blood flow ensures that oxygen and nutrients are efficiently delivered throughout the body, supporting overall tissue health and cardiovascular endurance. This is particularly beneficial for athletes seeking to boost performance and stamina, as well as individuals looking to maintain healthy blood pressure levels.

Furthermore, peptide bioregulators offer a holistic approach to cardiovascular well-being by reducing inflammation and supporting endothelial function. Their role in maintaining healthy cholesterol levels, preventing plaque formation, and enhancing metabolic processes contributes to long-term cardiovascular health. Additionally, their stress-reducing properties further safeguard heart health by mitigating the adverse effects of chronic stress. For health enthusiasts, fitness aficionados, busy professionals, and those interested in alternative medicine, integrating peptide bioregulators into their wellness regimen can be a natural and effective strategy for enhancing heart and vascular health.

CHAPTER 10

Hormonal Balance and Peptide Bioregulators

Maintaining hormonal balance is essential for overall health, vitality, and performance. Peptide bioregulators play a significant role in this process, influencing various hormone systems within the body. These small chains of amino acids are emerging as vital tools that help ensure hormones operate in harmony, supporting numerous bodily functions and promoting well-being.

This chapter delves into the multifaceted roles of peptide bioregulators in regulating crucial hormones such as insulin, testosterone, and growth hormone. Readers will gain insights into how these peptides impact glucose metabolism, muscle growth, energy levels, and mental clarity. Additionally, it explores the practical applications of peptide supplements to enhance athletic performance, cognitive function, and aging gracefully. By understanding the interplay between peptides and hormones, individuals can make informed decisions about their health, allowing for targeted and effective management of hormonal balance.

Regulating Hormone Levels

Peptide bioregulators are emerging as vital tools in the regulation of hormonal levels within the body. These peptides, small chains of amino acids, play crucial roles in balancing hormone systems, significantly impacting overall health, vitality, and performance. Understanding their functions provides valuable insights into maintaining a healthy hormonal equilibrium.

Various peptides have distinct roles when it comes to regulating important hormones such as insulin, testosterone, and growth hormone. For instance, peptides like insulinotropic polypeptides directly influence insulin secretion, which is paramount for glucose metabolism. Indeed, these peptides can enhance the body's response to insulin, ensuring blood sugar levels remain steady and reducing the risk of diabetes.

Testosterone-regulating peptides like Gonadotropin-Releasing Hormone (GnRH) are essential for both men and women. In men, proper testosterone levels support muscle mass, bone density, and libido. In women, balanced testosterone contributes to energy levels and reproductive health. Growth hormone-releasing peptides (GHRPs), on the other hand, stimulate the production of growth hormone, which is critical for tissue repair, muscle growth, and overall physical development.

Understanding these peptides allows readers to appreciate their importance in maintaining hormonal balance. Peptide bioregulators ensure that hormone levels do not fluctuate excessively, which could otherwise lead to various health issues such as fatigue, metabolic disorders, and decreased cognitive function. By recognizing the role of each peptide, individuals can better understand how to maintain their own hormonal health.

Moreover, knowledge of peptide roles empowers individuals to choose appropriate supplements for hormonal support. With a plethora of supplements available on the market, distinguishing between them becomes easier when one understands the specific functions of different peptides. For example, someone looking to improve their glucose metabolism might seek out insulinotropic peptide supplements, while an individual aiming to boost muscle recovery might opt for GHRPs.

Additionally, the integration of peptides into one's health regimen can be strategic. Athletes and fitness enthusiasts, for instance, might use tailored peptide supplements to enhance performance and recovery times. Meanwhile, busy professionals concerned about cognitive decline could benefit from peptides that support mental clarity and focus. This targeted approach ensures that supplementation is both effective and efficient, catering to the unique needs of every individual.

Hormone regulation by peptides significantly affects energy levels and overall well-being. When hormone levels are balanced, the body functions optimally. Insulin regulation via peptides ensures consistent energy supply by maintaining stable blood sugar levels. Conversely, imbalanced insulin can lead to energy crashes and fatigue, affecting daily productivity and performance.

Balanced testosterone levels, regulated by peptides, contribute to sustained energy, muscle strength, and endurance. For athletes, this balance is crucial for peak performance and quick recovery after intense physical activity. Similarly, balanced growth hormone levels mediated by peptides promote restful sleep, tissue repair, and muscle growth, all of which are essential for overall vitality.

Furthermore, hormonal balance aids in mental well-being. Cognitive functions like memory, focus, and mood are closely linked to hormone levels. Peptides that regulate cortisol, for example, help manage stress, leading to better mental clarity and stability. Balanced hormones reduce anxiety and depression, fostering a positive mental state.

A comprehensive understanding of how peptides influence hormone regulation underscores the interconnectedness of bodily systems. It highlights the holistic nature of health, where physical, mental, and emotional well-being are intertwined. Recognizing this interrelationship encourages a more integrated approach to personal health management.

In addition to their primary regulatory functions, peptides also offer preventive health benefits. Regular use of peptide bioregulators can mitigate potential hormonal imbalances before they manifest as serious health concerns. For instance, the early introduction of insulin-regulating peptides in individuals with prediabetic conditions can prevent the onset of full-blown diabetes.

The preventive aspect extends to age-related hormonal changes as well. As individuals age, natural hormone production declines, leading to various health issues. Peptide bioregulators can supplement diminished hormone levels, helping to maintain youthful vitality and delaying the impacts of aging. This proactive approach ensures sustained health and performance across the lifespan.

Moreover, the personalized nature of peptide supplementation aligns with modern trends in individualized healthcare. By tailoring peptide use to specific hormonal needs, individuals can achieve more effective and targeted health outcomes. Healthcare providers can assist in identifying the most suitable peptides based on personal health profiles, ensuring optimal results.

The practical applications of peptide bioregulators in everyday life are vast. For example, individuals facing chronic stress can benefit from cortisol-regulating peptides, enhancing their ability to cope with daily challenges. Similarly, those managing weight issues can use peptides that regulate hunger hormones, supporting healthier eating habits and weight control.

There is also growing interest in the role of peptides in anti-aging solutions. By regulating hormones associated with aging, such as growth hormone, peptides can slow down the aging process, preserving physical and mental faculties. This has significant implications for longevity and quality of life, making peptide bioregulation a key component of modern wellness strategies.

Hormonal Fluctuations and Aging

As individuals age, their hormonal levels can fluctuate dramatically, impacting both physical and mental health. Hormones are the body's chemical messengers, playing crucial roles in myriad bodily functions—from metabolism and growth to mood regulation and cognitive performance. Imbalances in these hormones can lead to a range of health issues, such as fatigue, weight gain, mood swings, reduced muscle mass, and cognitive decline. This is where peptide bioregulators come into play as powerful allies in mitigating age-related hormone imbalances.

Peptide bioregulators are short chains of amino acids that specifically target tissues and organs, guiding them toward optimal function. By promoting homeostasis, or balance within the body, these peptides help maintain hormonal stability even as we age. Research indicates that peptide bioregulators can effectively normalize the production and secretion of various hormones. For instance, they have been shown to influence the release of growth hormone, insulin, testosterone, and other critical hormones pivotal for maintaining youthful vitality.

Aging doesn't have to mean a natural and inevitable decline. Strategic supplementation with peptide bioregulators offers a way to counteract many of the adverse effects associated with getting older. Rather than accepting fatigue, decreased libido, and cognitive fog as part of the aging process, individuals can take proactive steps to support their hormonal health. Supplementing with peptide bioregulators can help maintain energy levels, enhance mood, and support muscle growth and recovery, providing a holistic approach to aging gracefully.

One substantial advantage of understanding how peptide bioregulators work is the practical application of this knowledge. For those looking to manage hormonal changes effectively, insights into peptide usage can be transformative. By incorporating specific peptides, individuals can tailor their health strategies to address their unique hormonal needs. This customization, a far cry from one-size-fits-all approaches, ensures more precise and effective management of age-related hormonal fluctuations.

Readers will discover that managing hormonal changes with peptide bioregulators resonates deeply with anyone aiming to maintain youthful vitality. Hormones like estrogen, progesterone, testosterone, and growth hormone naturally decrease with age, leading to symptoms often attributed to aging. But by leveraging peptide bioregulators, it's possible to stimulate the body's own production of these essential hormones or mimic their actions, thus mitigating the unsavory aspects of aging.

Taking charge of one's hormonal health requires not just an understanding of how peptides work but also a commitment to continuous learning and adaptation. As new research emerges, it becomes increasingly clear that targeted peptide therapy can offer profound benefits. Whether your goal is to improve physical performance, enhance mental clarity, or boost overall wellbeing, peptide bioregulators provide a promising path forward.

Moreover, practical ways to approach hormone-related aging issues often involve integrating peptide bioregulators into daily routines safely and effectively. This involves consulting healthcare providers knowledgeable about peptide therapy, starting with lower dosages, and tracking progress meticulously. Such practices are especially beneficial for busy professionals desiring enhanced focus and memory, athletes seeking improved performance, and health enthusiasts eager for longer, healthier lives.

The efficacy of peptide bioregulators in hormone balance extends beyond simple mitigation of decline. They represent a modern approach to aging, where maintaining peak physical and mental condition is within reach with appropriate intervention. The empowerment derived from using peptide bioregulators lies in their ability to provide concrete, science-backed solutions to age-related concerns, offering hope and tangible results.

Understanding the role and potential of peptide bioregulators equips readers with tools to make informed decisions about their health. It encourages a proactive stance toward aging, shifting the narrative from passive acceptance to active management. Peptides help bridge the gap between merely surviving and truly thriving during later years, fostering a sense of control and agency over one's health journey.

Natural Sources and Synthesis

Understanding the role that naturally produced peptides play in maintaining hormonal balance is crucial for anyone committed to improving their overall health and wellness. Peptides are short chains of amino acids that the body synthesizes and uses to signal various physiological processes, including hormone production and regulation. By understanding how lifestyle choices can influence endogenous peptide synthesis, individuals can make more informed decisions about their diets, exercise routines, and overall lifestyle.

Dietary choices have a profound impact on the body's ability to produce peptides. Consuming a balanced diet rich in proteins, vitamins, and minerals provides the building blocks necessary for peptide synthesis. Foods like lean meats, fish, eggs, dairy products, nuts, seeds, and legumes are particularly beneficial as they supply essential amino acids. Adequate hydration is also critical since water plays a key role in many biochemical reactions, including peptide formation.

Aside from diet, lifestyle factors such as regular physical activity greatly support the body's natural peptide production. Exercise prompts the release of growth hormone and other peptides that facilitate muscle repair, growth, and recovery. Regular aerobic activities like running, swimming, and cycling, coupled with strength training exercises, enhance the body's peptide synthesis capabilities. This symbiotic relationship between exercise and peptide production underscores the importance of maintaining an active lifestyle for optimal hormonal health.

Sleep and stress management also contribute significantly to endogenous peptide synthesis. Quality sleep enables the body to perform restorative functions, including the replenishment of peptides that regulate hormones like melatonin and cortisol. Conversely, chronic stress elevates cortisol levels, which can inhibit peptide production and disrupt hormonal balance. Therefore, incorporating relaxation techniques such as meditation, yoga, and deep-breathing exercises into daily routines can mitigate stress-induced hormonal imbalances by supporting healthy peptide levels.

Recognizing the relationship between simple lifestyle adjustments and hormonal health can empower readers to take proactive steps toward better well-being. Small changes, such as incorporating more protein-rich foods into meals, staying hydrated, engaging in regular physical activity, ensuring adequate sleep, and practicing stress management techniques, can collectively have a substantial impact on hormonal balance. These manageable adjustments can lead to improved energy levels, enhanced mental clarity, and overall better health.

This holistic approach suggests that dietary and lifestyle choices should not be viewed in isolation but rather as interdependent components of a comprehensive strategy for maintaining hormonal balance. Integrating peptide-rich foods and adopting habits that support the body's natural peptide production creates a synergistic effect that promotes overall health. For example, combining a nutritious diet with regular exercise and sufficient rest maximizes the benefits of each individual factor, leading to more efficient hormone regulation and better performance outcomes.

Moreover, understanding natural peptide production helps readers appreciate the body's intrinsic ability to maintain hormonal health and guides them in making informed decisions about their health routines. Recognizing that the body already possesses mechanisms for peptide synthesis encourages confidence in its natural healing and balancing capabilities. This awareness can motivate individuals to adopt lifestyle changes that enhance these natural processes rather than relying solely on external interventions.

For busy professionals interested in cognitive enhancement, natural peptide production offers pathways to improve focus, memory, and mental clarity. Peptides like brain-derived neurotrophic factor (BDNF) are crucial for brain health and cognitive function. Ensuring a diet rich in omega-3 fatty acids, antioxidants, and other nutrients supports the synthesis of such peptides. Combined with regular physical and mental exercises, these dietary choices foster an environment conducive to optimal brain function.

Athletes and fitness enthusiasts will find that supporting endogenous peptide synthesis through proper nutrition and exercise regimens enhances performance, muscle growth, and recovery times. Growth hormone-releasing peptides (GHRPs), for instance, play a vital role in muscle development and repair. A diet abundant in quality proteins and amino acids, alongside structured workout programs, can elevate GHRP levels naturally, thereby improving athletic performance and facilitating faster recovery.

Overall, recognizing natural peptide production encourages readers to make informed decisions about their health routines. By understanding the link between lifestyle choices and hormonal health, individuals are better positioned to take control of their well-being in a proactive and sustainable manner. The integration of dietary adjustments, regular physical activity, quality sleep, and effective stress management creates a robust framework for maintaining hormonal balance and achieving peak health.

As this chapter emphasizes, the body's natural ability to synthesize peptides and regulate hormones is influenced significantly by our daily choices. Emphasizing the importance of a holistic approach, where diet, exercise, sleep, and stress management are harmoniously integrated, offers a practical and empowering path to optimal health. Readers are encouraged to view these elements not as isolated tasks but as interconnected facets of a healthier, more balanced lifestyle.

Supporting Endocrine System

Peptide Bioregulators and the Endocrine System: A Vital Connection

The endocrine system plays a crucial role in maintaining various bodily functions through hormone production and secretion. It comprises several glands, including the pituitary, thyroid, adrenal glands, and pancreas, each of which secretes specific hormones that regulate processes like metabolism, growth, and mood. Understanding the structure and function of the endocrine system is the first step towards appreciating how peptide bioregulators can assist in maintaining hormonal health.

Hormones act as chemical messengers, traveling through the bloodstream to target organs and tissues, where they trigger specific physiological responses. For instance, insulin regulates glucose levels, while cortisol helps the body respond to stress. Disruptions in hormone production or secretion can lead to various health issues, such as diabetes, thyroid disorders, and adrenal insufficiency. Thus, the harmonious functioning of the endocrine system is essential for overall well-being.

Recognizing this intricate balance sets the stage for understanding the role of peptide bioregulators. Peptides are short chains of amino acids that can influence the behavior of cells and tissues. They interact with specific receptors on the surface of cells within different endocrine glands. For example, certain peptides can enhance insulin sensitivity, thereby supporting glucose metabolism. Others may influence the release of growth hormone, aiding in tissue repair and muscle growth.

The interaction between peptides and the endocrine system can be likened to a finely tuned orchestra. Each peptide has a unique role that contributes to the overall harmony. For example, thymic peptides support immune function, which indirectly influences hormonal health by reducing inflammatory stress on the adrenal glands. Similarly, pineal gland peptides can improve sleep quality by regulating melatonin production, which in turn supports the body's natural circadian rhythms.

Understanding these interactions provides a comprehensive view of health. The endocrine system does not operate in isolation; it is interconnected with other systems, such as the nervous and immune systems. Hormonal imbalances can affect mental health, immune response, and metabolic function. For instance, an overactive thyroid can lead to anxiety and weight loss, while insufficient cortisol can result in chronic fatigue and susceptibility to infections.

This interconnectedness emphasizes the importance of a holistic approach to health. Readers interested in wellness and longevity will find that supporting their endocrine system through peptide bioregulators can have far-reaching benefits. By maintaining hormonal balance, individuals can enhance their energy levels, cognitive function, and overall resilience. This is particularly relevant for athletes seeking improved performance and recovery, busy professionals aiming to boost focus and mental clarity, and those exploring anti-aging solutions.

Moreover, considering peptide support encourages proactive health management. Instead of addressing symptoms alone, individuals can target the underlying causes of hormonal imbalances. For example, peptides that promote the production of thyroid hormones can help manage hypothyroidism more effectively than symptomatic treatments alone. Similarly, peptides that modulate cortisol levels can offer a natural way to manage stress without relying solely on pharmaceutical interventions.

The impact of peptide bioregulators on metabolic health is another significant aspect. Metabolism is the process by which the body converts food into energy. Hormones like insulin and glucagon play pivotal roles in this process. Peptides that enhance insulin sensitivity or stimulate glucagon release can thus have a direct effect on energy levels and weight management.

For instance, peptide therapies can aid in muscle growth and recovery by stimulating the release of growth hormone and insulin-like growth factor (IGF). These peptides can be especially beneficial for fitness enthusiasts and athletes who require effective muscle repair and enhanced endurance. By optimizing these hormonal pathways, individuals can achieve better performance outcomes and quicker recovery times, which is vital for sustained physical activity.

Furthermore, the benefits of peptide bioregulators extend beyond physical health. Mental clarity and cognitive function are also influenced by hormonal balance. Neurotransmitters such as serotonin and dopamine, which affect mood and focus, are regulated by peptide interactions within the brain. Enhancing the production and function of these neurotransmitters can improve mental acuity and emotional stability, which is particularly beneficial for busy professionals or anyone dealing with cognitive decline.

In summary, peptide bioregulators offer a multifaceted approach to supporting the endocrine system. By influencing hormone production and secretion, these peptides help maintain the delicate balance required for optimal health. Their interactions with various glands underscore the interconnected nature of the endocrine system, emphasizing the need for a comprehensive view of health.

Impact on Stress Hormones

Peptides play a pivotal role in modulating the release of cortisol and other stress-related hormones, greatly influencing the body's stress response. Understanding how peptides interact with these hormones can unlock new strategies for managing stress, thus enhancing overall well-being.

Firstly, let's delve into the relationship between peptides and stress hormones. Peptides are short chains of amino acids that serve multiple functions in the body, including as signaling molecules that can influence the endocrine system. This system encompasses glands and organs responsible for hormone production and regulation. Cortisol, known as the "stress hormone," is produced by the adrenal glands and released during times of stress to provide the body with the necessary energy to respond to the challenge at hand. However, prolonged elevated levels of cortisol can have detrimental effects, such as impaired cognitive performance, suppressed immune function, and increased risk of chronic diseases like hypertension and diabetes.

Research has shown that certain peptides can help regulate the release of cortisol, thereby playing a crucial role in managing the body's stress response. For instance, the peptide corticotropin-releasing factor (CRF) influences the hypothalamus-pituitary-adrenal (HPA) axis, a central stress response system. By modulating this pathway, CRF and similar peptides can help maintain balanced cortisol levels, reducing the harmful impact of chronic stress. This interaction presents a powerful tool for integrating peptides into stress management strategies, which can be highly beneficial for individuals continually exposed to stressors.

Highlighting the importance of cortisol balance is essential for providing readers with actionable insights into using peptides for stress relief. Maintaining optimal cortisol levels not only mitigates the adverse effects of stress but also supports overall health and vitality. Balanced cortisol levels contribute to improved sleep quality, enhanced mood, better blood sugar regulation, and reduced inflammation. These benefits underscore the significance of keeping cortisol in check and demonstrate how peptide bioregulators can assist in achieving this balance.

Integrating peptides into daily routines for stress management requires a thorough understanding of their mechanisms and the right approach to supplementation. For example, peptides like adrenocorticotropic hormone (ACTH) stimulate the release of cortisol in response to stressors, but their activity must be regulated to prevent excessive cortisol production. On the other hand, peptides such as alpha-melanocyte-stimulating hormone (α-MSH) can counteract the negative effects of cortisol by promoting anti-inflammatory responses and enhancing tissue repair mechanisms.

Addressing the broader role of stress in health reveals how peptide supplementation can connect mental and physical well-being. Chronic stress not only affects emotional health but also has profound implications for physical fitness. Elevated cortisol levels can lead to muscle breakdown, impaired recovery from exercise, and decreased muscle growth. For athletes and fitness enthusiasts, managing cortisol through peptide supplementation can improve performance, enhance muscle recovery, and facilitate better adaptation to training regimens.

Furthermore, peptides' role in regulating stress hormones extends to cognitive health. Cortisol impacts brain function by affecting areas such as the hippocampus, which is critical for memory and learning. Excessive cortisol can impair cognitive abilities, leading to difficulties in focus, memory retention, and mental clarity. By modulating cortisol levels, peptides can help protect cognitive function, which is especially valuable for busy professionals seeking enhanced focus and productivity.

To effectively integrate peptides into stress management practices, it is crucial to adopt a holistic approach. This involves combining peptide supplementation with other stress-relief techniques such as mindfulness, exercise, and proper nutrition. For instance, incorporating peptides alongside adaptogenic herbs, which support the body's ability to adapt to stress, can amplify the benefits of both approaches. Mindfulness practices such as meditation and deep-breathing exercises can further enhance the stress-relieving effects of peptides by promoting relaxation and reducing the overall stress burden.

Additionally, peptides should be used wisely and tailored to individual needs. Not all peptides will suit everyone, and their effectiveness can vary depending on factors such as age, health status, and lifestyle. Consulting with healthcare professionals or specialists in peptide therapy can provide personalized guidance and ensure safe and effective use. Readers should be encouraged to start with lower dosages and gradually adjust based on their response, allowing them to find the most effective regimen for their specific needs.

This chapter has explored the significant influence of peptide bioregulators on maintaining hormonal balance, highlighting their impact on health, vitality, and performance. Understanding how peptides regulate hormones like insulin, testosterone, and growth hormone provides a clear path for enhancing overall well-being. By ensuring hormone levels remain stable, these peptides help prevent various health issues such as fatigue, metabolic disorders, and cognitive decline. Equipped with this knowledge, individuals can make informed choices about supplements that support their specific hormonal needs.

The practical applications of peptide bioregulators in everyday life are vast and diverse. Whether it's athletes seeking enhanced performance and recovery, busy professionals aiming to boost mental clarity, or health enthusiasts pursuing anti-aging solutions, peptides offer targeted and effective support. The integration of peptide bioregulators into daily routines represents a personalized approach to health management, emphasizing the interconnectedness of physical, mental, and emotional well-being. This comprehensive understanding empowers readers to take proactive steps in maintaining hormonal health, promoting a more balanced and vibrant lifestyle.

CHAPTER 11

Peptide Bioregulators in Holistic Medicine

Peptide bioregulators offer a promising addition to holistic medicine by enhancing the effectiveness of natural health practices. These small proteins are capable of fine-tuning various bodily functions, making them an appealing option for those seeking comprehensive health solutions. Peptides can interact with cellular processes to promote better absorption and utilization of nutrients, improve metabolic efficiency, and stimulate healing mechanisms. For individuals invested in optimizing their health through alternative therapies, the integration of peptide bioregulators holds significant potential.

This chapter will delve into how peptide bioregulators can complement traditional herbal treatments, amplify the benefits of acupuncture, and enhance stress-relief techniques like yoga. By exploring these synergies, readers will gain insights into how combining peptides with other natural therapies can lead to improved health outcomes. The discussion will include specific examples of how peptides can boost the bioavailability of herbal components, support pain management, and modulate stress responses, among other benefits. Whether you're looking to optimize your diet, improve athletic performance, or achieve mental clarity, this chapter provides evidence-based strategies for incorporating peptide bioregulators into your holistic health routine.

Integrating with Other Natural Therapies

The integration of peptide bioregulators within holistic and alternative health practices holds significant promise for enhancing overall health outcomes. By combining peptide bioregulators with various natural therapies, individuals can experience synergistic effects that promote well-being in diverse and complementary ways.

Peptide bioregulators are emerging as potent agents in the realm of traditional herbal treatments. These small proteins can interact with cellular mechanisms to regulate bodily functions, thereby augmenting the therapeutic effects of herbal remedies. For example, peptides can enhance the bioavailability of herbal components, allowing the body to absorb and utilize these substances more effectively. This synergistic relationship means that when used together, herbs and peptides can create a more robust healing response than either could achieve alone. Health enthusiasts who use herbal supplements for anti-aging, immune support, or general wellness might find their chosen therapies working more effectively when combined with specific peptides.

Another promising application is the integration of peptide therapy with acupuncture. Acupuncture has long been recognized for its ability to manage pain and reduce inflammation through the stimulation of specific points on the body. Peptides can complement this by targeting underlying biological pathways involved in pain and inflammation. For instance, certain peptides have anti-inflammatory properties that can reinforce the benefits of acupuncture. This holistic approach can be particularly beneficial for athletes dealing with sports injuries or busy professionals seeking relief from chronic pain. By combining these modalities, practitioners can offer a more comprehensive pain management strategy that addresses both symptoms and root causes.

Stress-relief techniques such as yoga also stand to gain from the incorporation of peptide bioregulators. Yoga emphasizes the connection between mind and body, promoting relaxation, mental clarity, and physical strength. Stress can disrupt these connections, leading to various mental and physical health problems. Peptides that influence stress hormones and neurotransmitters can amplify the benefits of yoga, helping to balance the body's stress response. For instance, peptides can modulate cortisol levels, reducing the impact of stress and enhancing relaxation induced by yoga practices. This combination creates a comprehensive mental wellness strategy that supports cognitive function, emotional balance, and physical resilience.

Tailoring peptide regimens to individual dietary habits offers another layer of personalized health optimization. Diet plays a crucial role in metabolic health, affecting everything from energy levels to weight management. Certain peptides can support metabolic functions by influencing processes like insulin sensitivity, fat metabolism, and appetite regulation. For individuals following specific dietary plans—whether for athletic performance, weight loss, or cognitive enhancement—customized peptide protocols can provide additional support, ensuring the diet yields maximum benefits. The fusion of tailored nutrition and peptide bioregulation can lead to improved metabolic efficiency and better overall health outcomes.

Synergies with Nutritional Interventions

In recent years, the interest in peptide bioregulators has surged, particularly within holistic and alternative health practices. These minute protein chains play a pivotal role in regulating various bodily functions, including metabolism, immune response, and cell repair. This section aims to elucidate how peptide bioregulators can effectively complement dietary changes or supplements, ultimately enhancing overall health outcomes.

One of the most compelling benefits of incorporating peptide bioregulators into dietary regimens is their potential to amplify nutrient absorption. Certain peptides can act as signaling molecules that instruct cells to optimize the uptake of essential nutrients. For instance, peptides like glutathione hold antioxidant properties that protect cells from oxidative stress while improving the absorption of vitamins such as Vitamin C and E. By ensuring that nutrients are more efficiently absorbed, these peptides make dietary interventions more effective, translating to better health and wellness outcomes for individuals.

The synergy between peptide bioregulators and nutrient-dense diets can potentially extend beyond mere nutrient absorption, contributing significantly to overall vitality. Nutrient-dense diets, rich in fruits, vegetables, lean proteins, and whole grains, provide the body with essential vitamins, minerals, and other vital compounds. When combined with peptide bioregulators, the body's ability to utilize these nutrients can be significantly enhanced. Peptides like collagen can improve gut health, aiding in the digestion and assimilation of nutrients, thereby boosting energy levels and promoting a sense of well-being. This combination can lead to improved physical health, faster recovery times, and enhanced mental clarity.

Another crucial aspect to consider is the customization of peptide regimens based on specific nutritional needs. The effectiveness of peptides can be maximized by tailoring them to an individual's unique dietary habits and health requirements. For example, a person deficient in certain minerals might benefit from peptides that enhance the absorption of those particular nutrients. Similarly, athletes might use specific peptides to support muscle recovery and growth, while older adults could benefit from peptides that promote bone health and cognitive function. This personalized approach ensures that the peptide regimen aligns closely with the individual's dietary intake, leading to optimized health outcomes.

When discussing guidelines, it becomes evident that consulting with healthcare practitioners to determine the appropriate type and dosage of peptide bioregulators is essential. Health professionals can provide tailored advice based on comprehensive assessments, ensuring the peptide supplements align with the individual's nutritional profile and health goals. This guidance is instrumental in preventing any adverse interactions between peptides and other ongoing treatments or supplements.

Moreover, combining peptide bioregulators with nutrition strategies aimed at enhancing metabolic functions can result in significant improvements in energy levels. Metabolism is the process through which our bodies convert food into energy. Peptide bioregulators can influence metabolic pathways, making energy production more efficient. For instance, peptides that stimulate mitochondrial function—the powerhouse of cells—can enhance energy output and reduce fatigue. Coupled with a balanced diet that supports metabolic health, these peptides can help individuals feel more energetic and focused throughout the day. Enhanced metabolic efficiency can also contribute to weight management, further driving home the importance of integrating peptides with dietary modifications.

To illustrate, consider the case of implementing peptide bioregulators alongside a Mediterranean diet, known for its abundance of healthy fats, proteins, fiber, and antioxidants. Peptides could potentially enhance the benefits of this diet by promoting better absorption of omega-3 fatty acids, crucial for brain health and anti-inflammatory responses. As a result, the combined approach not only supports the cardiovascular system but may also improve cognitive function and reduce the risk of chronic diseases.

Additionally, exploring the link between peptides and micronutrients can shed light on how these small proteins can bridge nutritional gaps. Micronutrients, although required in small amounts, play a significant role in maintaining health and preventing diseases. Peptides that aid in the absorption of micronutrients like zinc and magnesium can ensure that even minor dietary deficiencies are addressed, fostering a more robust immune system and healthier skin.

As we delve deeper into the practical applications, one cannot overlook the psychological benefits of this integrative approach. Improved nutrient absorption and metabolic function can have a cascading effect on mental health. Enhanced energy levels and physical well-being often correlate with better mood and cognitive capabilities. Thus, using peptides to supplement a nutrient-rich diet could indirectly mitigate issues like depression and anxiety, creating a holistic path to both physical and mental health improvement.

Mind-Body Practices

The integration of peptide bioregulators within holistic medicine offers a fascinating avenue to explore, especially when considering their synergy with practices like yoga and meditation. Peptide bioregulators are short chains of amino acids that influence various physiological processes. These bioregulators can significantly support the benefits gained from regular physical activity.

Regular physical activity, such as yoga, is known to improve flexibility, strength, and overall well-being. When combined with peptide bioregulators, these physiological benefits can be enhanced further. For instance, peptides are involved in muscle repair and growth, meaning they can help you recover more efficiently after your yoga sessions. This leads to improved performance over time, allowing for a more profound experience of the physical aspects of yoga.

Moreover, enhancements in cognitive function through peptide bioregulators can complement the mental clarity achieved through mindfulness practices. Meditation often focuses on achieving a state of mental calm and clarity. Certain peptides have been shown to enhance cognitive functions like memory, focus, and mental agility. By supporting brain health, peptides help deepen the mindfulness experience, making it easier to attain that desired state of mental tranquility.

Utilizing peptides along with stress-relief techniques creates a comprehensive strategy for mental wellness. Stress-relief techniques, including deep breathing exercises, meditation, and guided imagery, aim to reduce stress levels and promote a peaceful state of mind. Peptides, on the other hand, can regulate hormones such as cortisol, which is often elevated during stressful situations. By incorporating peptides into your stress-relief routine, you create a dual approach that not only targets stress at a psychological level but also addresses it biochemically. This holistic approach can lead to significant improvements in mental well-being.

Peptide bioregulators also play a crucial role in aiding recovery and building resilience in individuals participating in mind-body practices. Mind-body practices like yoga and meditation often require a high degree of physical and mental endurance. The wear and tear on muscles, joints, and mental faculties can be mitigated with peptide bioregulators. For example, specific peptides can aid in reducing inflammation and promoting tissue repair, which is essential for maintaining peak physical condition. Additionally, these peptides can support neural pathways associated with stress responses, building mental resilience over time.

Another interesting aspect is how peptide bioregulators can align with individualized treatment plans. Personalized treatment plans that include peptides could increase the effectiveness of holistic practices. Each individual's body responds differently to holistic treatments due to varying genetic makeups, lifestyles, and health conditions. Peptides can be tailored to meet these unique needs, enhancing the benefits derived from yoga and meditation. For instance, someone focusing on improving sleep quality might benefit from specific peptides that regulate sleep cycles and reduce anxiety.

The adaptability of peptide protocols allows customization for unique patient needs within various alternative health frameworks. Practitioners can modify peptide regimens to suit the specific requirements of their patients, whether they are athletes seeking quicker recovery times or busy professionals aiming to boost cognitive performance. This versatility ensures that peptide therapy can be integrated seamlessly into any holistic health practice, making it a valuable tool for practitioners.

Furthermore, the collaborative potential between peptide specialists and holistic practitioners could lead to improved interventions. Collaboration between experts in peptide therapy and those specializing in holistic practices can result in more effective and comprehensive treatment plans. This interdisciplinary approach enriches the scope of holistic medicine, providing patients with well-rounded care that addresses both their physical and mental health needs.

In practical terms, the integration of peptide bioregulators into holistic practices requires careful planning and monitoring. It is crucial to work closely with healthcare professionals who understand both peptide therapy and holistic practices. They can guide you in selecting the appropriate peptides, dosages, and combinations that will best support your individual health goals.

Case Studies and Success Stories

Integrating peptide bioregulators into holistic health practices has shown promising results in various settings. One notable application is the enhanced recovery from severe injuries when peptides are combined with physiotherapy. In these scenarios, patients who might have faced prolonged rehabilitation periods experienced faster healing times and improved mobility, demonstrating peptides' efficacy in recovery protocols. For instance, peptides promote cellular regeneration and tissue repair, which complement the physical exercises in physiotherapy aimed at restoring movement and strength. This synergy between peptides and physiotherapy provides a comprehensive approach to injury recovery, benefiting patients by reducing downtime and facilitating a quicker return to normal activities.

Another striking example is the improvement in memory retention observed through cognitive enhancement programs that integrate peptides with memory exercises. Memory decline is a common concern among busy professionals and aging individuals, impacting daily functioning and quality of life. Cognitive programs that include peptides have demonstrated significant benefits. Participants showed notable improvements in memory retention and cognitive speed, supporting the advantages of this integrated approach. Peptides can enhance neural connectivity and protect brain cells from age-related damage, thereby complementing memory exercises designed to stimulate cognitive function. This dual strategy offers a robust method to maintain mental clarity and prevent cognitive decline.

Athletes, constantly striving for peak performance, have also found benefits in incorporating peptides into their training routines. Significant strength and recovery improvements have been documented, making peptides an attractive option for fitness enthusiasts. By aiding muscle regeneration and reducing inflammation, peptides help athletes recover faster from intense workouts and injuries. This acceleration in recovery allows athletes to train more consistently and effectively. Furthermore, peptides can enhance protein synthesis, contributing to muscle growth and increased strength. These benefits make peptides a valuable addition to athletic training regimens, promoting overall better performance and resilience.

Cancer patients stand to gain substantially from utilizing peptide bioregulators alongside traditional treatments. While conventional cancer therapies like chemotherapy and radiation can be effective, they often come with severe side effects that deteriorate the patient's quality of life. Peptides can mitigate some of these side effects and improve patients' overall well-being. For instance, certain peptides can bolster the immune system, helping the body better tolerate aggressive cancer treatments. They can also aid in appetite stimulation and reduce fatigue, making day-to-day life more manageable for cancer patients. By integrating peptides with standard treatments, healthcare providers can offer a more holistic approach, addressing both the disease and the patient's overall health.

Insights into personalized care plans highlight the need for tailored therapies in achieving optimal results. Each individual's response to treatment can vary significantly, and personalizing peptide protocols ensures that the specific needs and conditions of patients are addressed. This customization maximizes therapeutic outcomes and minimizes potential side effects. For example, tailoring peptide regimens based on a patient's specific injury type, cognitive needs, athletic goals, or cancer treatment plan enables a more precise and effective intervention. This level of personalization underscores the necessity of collaboration between healthcare providers and peptide specialists to develop the most beneficial treatment strategies.

Integration in Holistic Protocols

Practitioners aiming to incorporate peptide bioregulators into holistic health protocols must first recognize the unique benefits of personalized treatment plans that include these peptides. Unlike one-size-fits-all approaches, personalized plans tailor interventions based on individual patient needs, enhancing the effectiveness of holistic practices. For example, a health enthusiast interested in anti-aging might benefit from peptides that support skin regeneration and cellular repair. This customization ensures that each patient receives the most appropriate and effective treatment for their specific health goals.

The adaptability of peptide protocols is another significant advantage. Peptides can be adjusted in response to changes in a patient's condition or health objectives. A fitness enthusiast looking to improve muscle growth and recovery times might start with peptides designed to boost protein synthesis. As their training regimens evolve, so too can their peptide protocols, ensuring continuous alignment with their changing needs. This flexibility makes peptides an invaluable tool in the hands of skilled holistic practitioners, who can modify treatments as required for optimal outcomes.

Collaboration between peptide specialists and holistic practitioners could lead to improved interventions. Holistic practitioners often have extensive knowledge in various natural therapies but may lack specific expertise in peptide bioregulation. By working closely with peptide specialists, they can develop more comprehensive and effective treatment protocols. For instance, a holistic practitioner treating a busy professional concerned about cognitive decline might collaborate with a peptide specialist to integrate peptides known for enhancing focus, memory, and mental clarity into their wellness plan. Such collaborative efforts can result in well-rounded and highly effective health interventions.

Integration strategies can be tailored to different alternative health frameworks for optimal outcomes. Holistic medicine encompasses a wide range of practices, from traditional Chinese medicine to Ayurveda. Each framework has its own set of principles and methods, which means that the integration of peptides must be handled thoughtfully. In Ayurveda, for example, balancing doshas is crucial. Peptide regimens can be designed to complement this balance, perhaps by using peptides that promote detoxification and rejuvenation in line with Ayurvedic cleansing protocols. Similarly, in traditional Chinese medicine, peptides can be integrated to enhance the flow of qi and improve overall energy balance.

To ensure successful incorporation of peptides into holistic protocols, practitioners should consider several guidelines. First, they should conduct thorough assessments to identify the specific needs and conditions of each patient. This helps in creating a targeted peptide regimen that aligns with the individual's health goals. Additionally, continuous monitoring and adjustments are essential. Regular follow-ups allow practitioners to evaluate the effectiveness of peptide protocols and make necessary modifications. This ongoing process ensures that patients receive the most beneficial and up-to-date treatments.

Moreover, education and training are vital for holistic practitioners venturing into peptide therapy. Understanding the science behind peptide bioregulators, their mechanisms of action, and potential side effects is crucial. Training programs and workshops on peptide therapy can equip practitioners with the knowledge and skills needed to effectively integrate peptides into their practice. This not only enhances their competency but also boosts patient confidence in their holistic care provider.

Integrating peptide bioregulators with other natural therapies offers promising advancements in holistic health practices. By combining peptides with herbal treatments, acupuncture, and stress-relief techniques like yoga and meditation, individuals can achieve enhanced health outcomes.

Peptides improve bioavailability, support pain management, and regulate stress responses, creating a more effective and comprehensive approach to wellness. Such synergy not only augments the benefits of traditional treatments but also addresses both physical and mental health needs, making it easier for individuals to reach their wellness goals.

Furthermore, personalized peptide regimens tailored to specific dietary habits and health objectives provide an additional layer of optimization. Customizing peptides based on individual needs ensures maximum effectiveness, particularly when combined with nutrient-dense diets or nutritional interventions. Addressing unique health conditions through specialized peptide protocols boosts energy levels, improves cognitive functions, and enhances physical resilience. The collaboration between healthcare professionals and holistic practitioners is essential for safely integrating these therapies, ensuring that peptide use aligns well with existing treatments and promotes overall well-being.

CHAPTER 12

Fitness and Recovery

F itness and recovery are pivotal aspects of maintaining optimal health and achieving peak performance in physical activities. This chapter delves into the role of peptide bioregulators in aiding physical recovery and muscle repair, specifically focusing on how these compounds can enhance overall wellbeing by speeding up recovery times and reducing muscle soreness. By comprehending the functions and benefits of peptide bioregulators, individuals can make informed choices to support their fitness routines and recovery processes.

Throughout this chapter, readers will explore the scientific mechanisms by which peptide bioregulators operate. The discussion includes how these peptides promote faster muscle repair through cellular regeneration, manage post-exercise inflammation efficiently, and ensure effective nutrient delivery to recovering muscles. Furthermore, the chapter highlights the importance of hormonal balance in muscle recovery and describes how peptide bioregulators influence this balance. By understanding these facets, health enthusiasts, athletes, busy professionals, and those interested in holistic health approaches can appreciate the value of incorporating peptide bioregulators into their fitness and wellness regimens.

Speeds Up Recovery Time

Peptide bioregulators play a crucial role in expediting the recovery process after strenuous exercise. Let's delve into the scientific mechanisms through which these powerful compounds operate, starting with their ability to promote faster muscle repair. When you exert your muscles during a workout, micro-tears occur within the muscle fibers. Your body must repair these tears to build stronger and more resilient muscles. Peptide bioregulators facilitate this repair by promoting cellular regeneration. These peptides help stimulate the production of new cells, aiding in the quick replacement of damaged ones. This cell turnover is essential for efficient muscle repair, allowing athletes and fitness enthusiasts to recover quicker and resume their training routines without prolonged downtime.

Managing inflammation is another critical aspect of post-exercise recovery where peptide bioregulators come into play. After intense physical activity, inflammation is a natural response that helps in the healing process. However, excessive or prolonged inflammation can lead to discomfort and delayed recovery. Peptide bioregulators help manage this inflammation by regulating inflammatory pathways. They act on specific cytokines and other inflammatory mediators, reducing the inflammatory response without completely shutting it down. This balance ensures that the necessary repair processes can continue while minimizing pain and discomfort, making it easier to get back to physical activities sooner.

Effective nutrient delivery is fundamental to muscle recovery, and peptide bioregulators significantly enhance blood flow to tissues. Improved circulation means that oxygen and nutrients are delivered more efficiently to the recovering muscles. Oxygen is vital for the cellular respiration process, which generates the energy needed for muscle repair. Moreover, nutrients like amino acids, vitamins, and minerals are crucial building blocks for new muscle tissue. By enhancing blood flow, peptide bioregulators ensure that these essential components reach the muscle cells promptly, facilitating quicker recovery and reduced muscle soreness.

Support for hormonal balance is yet another way peptide bioregulators optimize muscle repair processes. Hormones like testosterone and growth hormone are pivotal in muscle growth and repair. Peptides can influence the endocrine system to maintain optimal levels of these hormones, thus supporting anabolic processes that build and repair muscle tissue. For instance, certain peptides can stimulate the release of growth hormone, which enhances protein synthesis and promotes the formation of new muscle fibers. This hormonal support accelerates the repair process, ensuring that muscles recovery efficiently.

Athletes who incorporate peptide bioregulators into their recovery regimen often report feeling less muscle soreness and fatigue post-exercise. This feedback aligns with the scientific understanding of how these peptides function. By managing inflammation, enhancing nutrient delivery, and supporting hormonal balance, peptide bioregulators create an environment conducive to rapid muscle recovery. This means athletes can train more consistently and effectively, leading to better overall performance and reduced risk of overuse injuries.

It's also worth noting that peptide bioregulators are naturally occurring compounds, often derived from animal sources or synthesized to mimic natural peptides in the body. Their use offers a more holistic approach to recovery compared to synthetic drugs, which may have unwanted side effects. For those interested in alternative medicine and wellness supplements, peptide bioregulators provide a natural option to enhance recovery and overall fitness.

The interaction between peptide bioregulators and the body's endogenous systems underscores their effectiveness. By working synergistically with the body's natural processes, these peptides ensure a balanced approach to muscle repair and recovery. This symbiotic relationship not only speeds up recovery but also contributes to long-term muscle health and resilience.

Incorporating peptide bioregulators into a fitness routine requires an understanding of the timing and dosage for optimal results. Generally, these peptides are administered through injections or oral supplements. It's important to follow recommended guidelines to avoid potential adverse effects and to maximize benefits. Consulting with a healthcare professional is advisable before starting any new supplement regimen, especially for individuals with underlying health conditions or those taking other medications.

Enhanced Muscle Repair

Peptide bioregulators have gained attention in the fitness and recovery community due to their ability to enhance muscle repair. By promoting cellular regeneration, these compounds accelerate tissue repair processes, essential for anyone engaged in regular physical activity. When muscles undergo stress during exercise, minor injuries are inevitable. The body's natural response is to repair these tissues, making them stronger. Peptide bioregulators can expedite this process by enhancing the production of proteins vital for cell structure and function, thus supporting faster muscle fiber repair.

Reducing downtime between workouts is another significant advantage offered by peptide bioregulators. Consistent training is crucial for athletes aiming to achieve their fitness goals. However, the time required for recovery often limits the frequency and intensity of workouts. Peptide bioregulators mitigate this challenge by fostering quicker muscle recovery. This allows athletes to return to their routines sooner and reduce breaks between sessions. With reduced downtime, individuals can maintain a steady training regimen, which is pivotal for continual improvement in strength and performance.

Moreover, these bioregulators play a crucial role in increasing circulation throughout the body, which is fundamental for muscle recovery and repair. Enhanced blood flow ensures adequate oxygen delivery to muscles, which is necessary for cellular respiration and energy production. Efficient circulation also helps remove metabolic waste products that accumulate during intense physical activities. These waste products, if not promptly cleared, can contribute to muscle fatigue and soreness. By improving circulation, peptide bioregulators help cleanse the muscle tissue of these byproducts, facilitating a quicker recovery process.

Supporting optimal hormonal levels is another critical function of peptide bioregulators in muscle repair. Hormones such as testosterone and growth hormone significantly influence muscle synthesis and repair. Peptide bioregulators aid in maintaining balanced hormonal levels, ensuring that the body has the right signals for effective muscle recovery. For instance, growth hormone promotes the development and repair of muscle fibers, while testosterone enhances protein synthesis in muscle cells. By regulating these hormones, peptide bioregulators enhance the body's natural ability to repair and build muscle tissue.

The promotion of cellular regeneration for quicker tissue repair is one of the primary ways peptide bioregulators aid in muscle recovery. Cellular regeneration involves the replacement of damaged or old cells with new ones, ensuring the maintenance of healthy tissue. Peptide bioregulators stimulate the production of specific proteins that are integral to cell growth and repair. This leads to more efficient healing of microtears caused by strenuous exercises, allowing muscles to recover faster and more effectively. The accelerated repair not only reduces recovery time but also strengthens the muscles, making them more resilient to future stress.

In addition to reducing downtime and promoting cellular regeneration, peptide bioregulators help maintain consistent training schedules. Frequent breaks or prolonged recovery periods can disrupt an athlete's routine, affecting their overall progress. Peptide bioregulators minimize these interruptions by speeding up the recovery process, enabling athletes to engage in regular, high-intensity training without the prolonged rest periods typically needed after intense workouts. This consistency is essential for building endurance, strength, and overall physical performance.

Furthermore, the increase in circulation facilitated by peptide bioregulators ensures better oxygenation of the tissues. Oxygen is a critical component in the production of adenosine triphosphate (ATP), the energy currency of cells. Adequate oxygen supply through improved blood circulation helps sustain ATP levels, providing muscles with the energy required for repair and growth. Additionally, enhanced circulatory function aids in the delivery of nutrients, such as amino acids and glucose, which are vital for muscle repair and recovery. This comprehensive support system ensures that muscles receive all the necessary elements for efficient recovery and strength development.

Optimal hormonal balance is fundamental for muscle repair, and peptide bioregulators contribute significantly to this aspect. Hormonal imbalances can impede muscle recovery and lead to various health issues. Peptide bioregulators ensure that hormones related to muscle repair and growth are maintained at ideal levels. This not only promotes effective repair of muscle tissue but also supports overall well-being. Balanced hormonal levels contribute to better energy levels, mood stability, and enhanced physical performance, creating a conducive environment for continuous fitness progress.

Promoting quicker tissue repair through cellular regeneration is a cornerstone of how peptide bioregulators improve muscle recovery. By stimulating the production of proteins and other molecules essential for cell growth and repair, they ensure that damaged muscle fibers are swiftly and efficiently restored. This rapid repair mechanism minimizes muscle soreness and stiffness, common after intense workouts, allowing athletes to resume their activities with minimal discomfort. The quicker repair time provided by peptide bioregulators thus becomes a valuable asset for anyone seeking to optimize their physical performance and recovery.

Reducing downtime between workouts is particularly beneficial for busy professionals and athletes striving to maximize their training efficiency. Peptide bioregulators allow for shorter recovery periods, enabling more frequent and consistent workouts. This continuity in training not only accelerates progress but also enhances motivation and commitment. Knowing that recovery times will be brief and manageable encourages individuals to push their limits and engage more fully in their fitness routines, leading to greater overall achievements in their physical endeavors.

Enhancing circulation through the use of peptide bioregulators is instrumental in muscle recovery. Proper circulation ensures that muscles receive a steady supply of oxygen and nutrients required for repair and growth. It also facilitates the removal of lactic acid and other metabolic waste products that accumulate during exercise, reducing the likelihood of cramps and soreness. Enhanced blood flow supports overall cardiovascular health, contributing to better fitness outcomes and faster recovery times. By optimizing circulation, peptide bioregulators provide a holistic approach to muscle repair and overall physical well-being.

Supporting optimal hormonal levels cannot be overstated when discussing muscle repair. Hormones like insulin, cortisol, and growth factors play a critical role in how the body rebuilds muscle tissue post-exercise. Peptide bioregulators help maintain these hormones at levels conducive to muscle repair and growth. This hormonal support ensures that the body responds effectively to the demands of physical activity, promoting faster recovery and increased muscle mass. For athletes and fitness enthusiasts, this means improved performance, greater muscle definition, and enhanced overall fitness.

Reduction of Inflammation

Peptide bioregulators have emerged as a promising solution for managing inflammation after intense physical activity. These small chains of amino acids play a crucial role in reducing post-workout inflammation, enabling athletes and fitness enthusiasts to enhance their overall fitness levels. Post-workout inflammation is a natural response to muscle strain and exertion, but if left unmanaged, it can lead to discomfort, delayed recovery, and even injuries.

One of the primary benefits of peptide bioregulators is their ability to manage post-workout inflammation effectively. By modulating the body's inflammatory response, these peptides help reduce the swelling and redness often associated with intense exercise. This reduction in inflammation accelerates the healing process, allowing muscles to repair more quickly and efficiently. The quicker recovery time ultimately enables individuals to return to their workout routines sooner, thereby maintaining their fitness momentum.

Less inflammation also means less discomfort. Muscles that are not inflamed are less likely to be sore and tender, which significantly reduces post-exercise pain. This alleviation of discomfort is particularly beneficial for those who engage in regular, strenuous workouts, as it minimizes the downtime needed for recovery. Moreover, by mitigating pain, peptide bioregulators make the entire exercise experience more enjoyable, encouraging individuals to stick to their fitness routines without the dread of post-workout soreness.

Effective inflammation management through peptide bioregulators also plays a pivotal role in reducing the risk of injuries. When inflammation is kept in check, the likelihood of overuse injuries decreases. Overuse injuries often occur when individuals push their bodies too hard without giving sufficient time for recovery. By accelerating the recovery process and reducing inflammation, peptide bioregulators allow muscles to heal properly, thus preventing strains, sprains, and other common exercise-related injuries. This protective effect is especially crucial for athletes who consistently challenge their physical limits.

Furthermore, controlling inflammation is essential for improving long-term adherence to workout routines. Pain and discomfort are significant barriers to consistent exercise, often causing people to abandon their fitness goals. By using peptide bioregulators to manage inflammation and ease post-workout pain, individuals are more likely to stay committed to their exercise programs. This consistency is key to achieving long-term fitness and health objectives. Regular physical activity, supported by reduced inflammation and pain, contributes to overall wellness, including improved cardiovascular health, better weight management, and enhanced mental clarity.

In addition to the physiological benefits, there is a psychological advantage to managing inflammation with peptide bioregulators. The anticipation of post-exercise pain can be a significant deterrent for many individuals. Knowing that they have a tool to combat inflammation and reduce soreness can boost morale and motivation. This positive mindset further reinforces the habit of regular exercise, creating a cycle of continuous improvement and well-being.

The effectiveness of peptide bioregulators in managing inflammation can be attributed to their action at the cellular level. These peptides interact with specific receptors in the body to regulate the production of pro-inflammatory cytokines. By inhibiting these inflammatory molecules, peptide bioregulators prevent excessive inflammation while still allowing the necessary immune response for muscle repair. This targeted approach ensures that the body can recover optimally without the detrimental effects of chronic inflammation.

Moreover, peptide bioregulators offer a natural method of inflammation management. Unlike non-steroidal anti-inflammatory drugs (NSAIDs) that can cause side effects like gastrointestinal issues and cardiovascular risks, peptide bioregulators work harmoniously with the body's natural processes. This makes them a safer alternative for long-term use, providing sustained benefits without adverse effects.

It's important to note that the benefits of peptide bioregulators extend beyond just managing acute post-workout inflammation. They also play a role in mitigating chronic inflammation, which is linked to various health conditions such as arthritis, heart disease, and metabolic syndrome. By incorporating peptide bioregulators into their regimen, individuals not only enhance their recovery from exercise but also support their overall health and longevity.

For busy professionals, managing inflammation effectively is crucial, as it allows them to balance their demanding schedules with their fitness pursuits. The reduction in pain and discomfort means less distraction and more focus on work and personal commitments. Additionally, the improved recovery times enable them to maximize their limited workout windows, achieving their fitness goals without compromising their professional responsibilities.

Reduces Muscle Soreness

Peptide bioregulators have emerged as a fascinating subject in the field of fitness and recovery. One of their most notable benefits is the mitigation of muscle soreness following strenuous physical activity. Understanding this can be a game changer for individuals who are deeply involved in regular physical training or for those new to exercise. By focusing on how peptide bioregulators alleviate delayed onset muscle soreness (DOMS), provide natural pain-relieving properties, and enhance motivation and long-term adaptations, we can see just how valuable these compounds are.

Let's begin with delayed onset muscle soreness or DOMS, a common result of intense workouts. DOMS typically manifests 24 to 72 hours post-exercise and can be a barrier to continuous training schedules. Peptide bioregulators play a crucial role in reducing this soreness, allowing for more frequent and consistent exercise routines. When muscles are less sore, athletes and fitness enthusiasts can train more regularly without taking prolonged breaks for recovery. This consistency is essential as it leads to better overall performance and quicker achievement of fitness goals. Research suggests that by targeting specific peptides in the body, it's possible to enhance the repair processes at the cellular level, thus mitigating the effects of DOMS more effectively than traditional methods.

Next is the natural pain-relieving property of peptide bioregulators. Unlike synthetic painkillers, which often come with side effects and the risk of dependency, peptide bioregulators offer a more holistic approach. These bioactive peptides can interact with the body's own pain management systems, providing relief without disrupting other bodily functions. The natural relief from discomfort not only makes exercising more pleasant but also reduces reliance on pharmaceutical interventions. For instance, peptides like BPC-157 have been shown in studies to accelerate the healing of tendons and ligaments, which indirectly relieves the pain caused by microtears during intense physical activities. This allows the user to focus on their workouts without the constant interruption of pain or the concern of causing further injury.

When soreness is reduced, there's a notable improvement in motivation and mental outlook. Exercise-induced muscle pain can often lead to discouragement, especially among beginners or those returning after a long hiatus. Knowing that there are supportive measures like peptide bioregulators to ease this journey can significantly boost morale. A positive mind frame is not only beneficial for maintaining regular physical activity but also for setting and achieving higher fitness goals. The psychological benefits can't be overstated; being free from pain increases the enjoyment of workouts and fosters a stronger commitment to an active lifestyle. This improved outlook can also reduce stress levels, contributing to overall well-being and enhanced workout performance.

Finally, the long-term benefits of using peptide bioregulators are particularly noteworthy. Consistent use leads to better adaptations and greater fitness capacity over time. By enabling continuous training and quick recovery, the body undergoes more substantial improvements in strength, endurance, and flexibility. This aspect is vital for both professional athletes aiming for peak performance and regular individuals striving for optimal health. The reduced wear and tear on muscles and quicker recovery times mean fewer injuries and more efficient training sessions. Over time, this results in more pronounced muscle definition, increased muscle mass, and overall better physical condition.

In addition to muscle-centric advantages, peptide bioregulators contribute to a holistic enhancement of bodily functions, promoting balance and harmony throughout various systems. This comprehensive benefit ensures that while muscles recover and strengthen, other areas such as joint health, cardiovascular efficiency, and even cognitive function are supported.

For example, peptides like TB-500 have been shown to promote cell migration and repair, which is beneficial not only for muscles but for overall tissue repair. This broader application means that users experience a more integrative form of recovery, making peptide bioregulators a versatile choice for anyone looking to improve their physical health.

Furthermore, incorporating peptide bioregulators into a fitness regime can act as a preventive measure against overtraining syndrome, a common issue faced by dedicated athletes. Overtraining can lead to persistent fatigue, decreased performance, and higher susceptibility to injuries. By optimizing recovery through the targeted action of peptide bioregulators, the risks associated with overtraining are minimized, ensuring sustained progress and peak performance.

Improved Circulation

Peptide bioregulators, small protein molecules that influence the behavior of cells and tissues, play a crucial role in enhancing blood flow and nutrient delivery during physical recovery. This enhanced circulation is fundamental for several reasons, primarily due to its impact on muscle repair and recovery, nutrient transport, elimination of metabolic waste, and overall fitness performance.

One of the key benefits of improved blood flow through peptide bioregulators is increased oxygenation of muscle tissues. Oxygen is essential for the production of adenosine triphosphate (ATP), the primary energy currency of cells. When muscles are adequately oxygenated, they can produce more ATP, which is necessary for repairing damaged tissues and promoting cellular regeneration. An increase in oxygen supply helps reduce the time required for muscle recovery, as it enables cells to work efficiently in the healing process. Athletes often experience quicker recovery times, allowing them to return to training faster and maintain their fitness levels.

Moreover, peptide bioregulators enhance nutrient transport to tissues. Nutrients such as amino acids, vitamins, and minerals are vital for muscle repair and growth. When these nutrients are delivered more effectively to muscle tissues, it accelerates the healing process. Enhanced nutrient transport ensures that muscle fibers receive the building blocks they need to recover from strenuous activity. For example, proteins are essential for repairing microtears in muscle fibers caused by intense workouts. Peptide bioregulators facilitate the efficient delivery of these proteins, speeding up recovery and promoting muscle growth.

The process of cellular metabolism generates waste products, including lactic acid and carbon dioxide. Accumulation of these waste products can lead to muscle fatigue and soreness, hindering recovery. Faster elimination of metabolic waste is another significant advantage of enhanced circulation facilitated by peptide bioregulators. By improving blood flow, these peptides help remove waste products more rapidly from muscle tissues. This not only reduces muscle soreness but also prevents prolonged discomfort, enabling individuals to resume their physical activities sooner.

Improved circulation through peptide bioregulators supports overall better fitness performance. Consistent and adequate blood flow ensures that all body tissues receive the oxygen and nutrients they require for optimal function. Enhanced blood circulation means that muscles are well-nourished and capable of performing at their best. This is particularly beneficial for athletes who demand peak performance from their bodies. With improved blood flow, they can train harder, recover faster, and achieve better results in their respective sports.

Increased oxygenation, nutrient transport, and waste removal collectively provide a comprehensive approach to muscle recovery. When muscles receive sufficient oxygen, nutrients, and efficient waste clearance, they can repair themselves more effectively. This holistic approach to recovery not only reduces downtime between workouts but also minimizes the risk of injuries related to muscle fatigue and overuse.

It is important to understand the mechanism behind how peptide bioregulators enhance blood flow. These peptides influence the release of nitric oxide, a potent vasodilator that relaxes blood vessels and allows for increased blood flow. Nitric oxide widens blood vessels, reducing resistance and enabling a greater volume of blood to reach muscle tissues. As a result, oxygen and nutrients are delivered more efficiently, while waste products are removed more rapidly. This vasodilation effect is particularly useful for athletes who experience muscle fatigue and soreness after intense training sessions. By increasing blood flow to fatigued muscles, peptide bioregulators aid in quicker recovery and reduced discomfort.

While the benefits of peptide bioregulators on blood flow and nutrient delivery are significant, it is also essential to consider their long-term effects on overall health and wellness. Regular use of peptide bioregulators can promote sustained improvements in circulation, leading to better cardiovascular health. Improved blood flow supports not only muscle recovery but also the function of vital organs, contributing to overall longevity and well-being. For individuals interested in anti-aging solutions, peptide bioregulators offer a natural way to support the body's regenerative processes and maintain youthful vitality.

Additionally, peptide bioregulators can be an excellent addition to holistic health approaches. Those who prefer alternative medicine and wellness supplements may find peptide bioregulators align with their health goals. By enhancing the body's natural ability to heal and recover, these peptides support a balanced and integrated approach to wellness. They can be incorporated into a broader regimen that includes proper nutrition, regular exercise, and other complementary therapies.

Athletes and fitness enthusiasts, in particular, stand to gain significantly from the use of peptide bioregulators. The ability to recover quickly from workouts and reduce muscle soreness enables them to train more consistently and effectively. This consistency is key to achieving long-term fitness goals and improving athletic performance. Moreover, by reducing the risk of injuries associated with overtraining and muscle fatigue, peptide bioregulators help athletes maintain peak condition throughout their competitive seasons.

For busy professionals concerned about cognitive decline, the benefits of peptide bioregulators extend beyond physical recovery. Improved circulation enhances the delivery of oxygen and nutrients to the brain, supporting cognitive function and mental clarity. By ensuring that the brain receives adequate oxygen, peptide bioregulators may help improve focus, memory, and overall cognitive performance. This can be particularly valuable for individuals who need to stay sharp and focused in demanding work environments.

This chapter has discussed the vital role of peptide bioregulators in aiding physical recovery and muscle repair. These compounds work by promoting cellular regeneration, managing inflammation, enhancing nutrient delivery, and supporting hormonal balance. This multifaceted approach helps to speed up recovery time and reduces muscle soreness, allowing individuals to maintain consistent training routines and improve overall performance.

For athletes and fitness enthusiasts, incorporating peptide bioregulators offers a natural and holistic method to optimize recovery processes. Enhanced circulation ensures that muscles receive the necessary oxygen and nutrients, facilitating quicker repair and reducing downtime. Furthermore, peptide bioregulators provide an alternative to synthetic drugs, aligning with those who prefer wellness supplements. By working synergistically with the body, these peptides support long-term muscle health and resilience, making them a valuable addition to any fitness or wellness regimen.

CHAPTER 13

Peptide Bioregulators and Mental Health

Peptide bioregulators have drawn significant interest for their potential to improve mental health by reducing anxiety and depression while enhancing emotional stability. As naturally occurring molecules that play a crucial role in physiological processes, peptide bioregulators can influence the brain's functioning in several ways. This chapter delves into how these molecules interact with key neurotransmitters like serotonin and dopamine, which are essential for mood regulation.

The chapter will also explore how peptide bioregulators modulate the stress response, thereby helping to manage symptoms of anxiety and emotional instability. Additionally, it examines the role of chronic inflammation in contributing to mood disorders and how peptides can mitigate this inflammation to promote better mental health. Finally, the discussion will highlight the growing body of clinical evidence supporting the use of peptide bioregulators and provide insights and examples from both research studies and real-world applications. This comprehensive examination aims to equip readers with a well-rounded understanding of how peptide bioregulators can be integrated into mental wellness strategies.

Reducing Anxiety and Depression

Peptide bioregulators have garnered attention for their potential impact on mental health, specifically in mitigating symptoms of anxiety and depression. These naturally occurring molecules are crucial in maintaining physiological processes and can influence various aspects of brain function. This section delves into how peptide bioregulators affect neurotransmitter regulation, stress response modulation, inflammation reduction, and the clinical evidence supporting their use.

One of the primary ways peptide bioregulators can help manage anxiety and depression is through the regulation of neurotransmitters such as serotonin and dopamine. These neurotransmitters play a pivotal role in mood regulation and emotional well-being. Serotonin is often referred to as the "feel-good" neurotransmitter because it contributes to feelings of happiness and relaxation. Dopamine, on the other hand, is associated with motivation, pleasure, and reward. An imbalance in either of these chemicals can lead to mood disorders. By influencing the production, release, and reuptake of these neurotransmitters, peptide bioregulators can help restore balance and improve mood. For instance, certain peptides have been shown to increase serotonin levels, which can help alleviate symptoms of depression and promote a sense of calm.

Stress response modulation is another critical area where peptide bioregulators exert their beneficial effects. The body's stress response is a complex system involving the release of hormones such as cortisol and adrenaline. While these hormones are essential for survival, chronic stress can lead to prolonged exposure to these chemicals, resulting in anxiety and other stress-related disorders. Peptide bioregulators can help modulate this stress response by influencing the hypothalamic-pituitary-adrenal (HPA) axis, which controls the release of stress hormones. By doing so, they can ease anxiety symptoms during stressful situations and promote emotional stability. For example, some peptides can reduce cortisol levels, thereby decreasing the overall stress burden on the body and mind.

Inflammation has been increasingly recognized as a contributing factor to mood disorders, including anxiety and depression. Chronic inflammation can disrupt normal brain function and lead to the development of depressive symptoms. Peptide bioregulators can help reduce inflammation, thus preventing the decline in mood associated with inflammatory conditions. They achieve this by modulating the activity of immune cells and reducing the production of pro-inflammatory cytokines, which are signaling molecules that promote inflammation. By lowering inflammation, peptide bioregulators not only support physical health but also contribute to improved mental well-being. For instance, studies have shown that certain peptides can decrease levels of inflammatory markers in the blood, leading to reduced symptoms of depression and anxiety.

The growing body of clinical evidence supports the use of peptide bioregulators in alleviating anxiety and depression. Emerging research, including both animal and human studies, highlights the potential therapeutic benefits of these molecules. For example, clinical trials have demonstrated that certain peptides can effectively reduce anxiety symptoms in patients with generalized anxiety disorder. Similarly, research has shown that peptides can improve mood and decrease depressive symptoms in individuals with major depressive disorder. These findings are backed by case studies and anecdotal reports from individuals who have experienced significant improvements in their mental health after using peptide bioregulators. As more research is conducted, the understanding of how these peptides work and their potential applications in mental health management will continue to expand.

Neurotransmitter Regulation

Peptide bioregulators are emerging as a significant tool in the realm of mental health, particularly for their role in balancing neurotransmitter levels. Neurotransmitters like serotonin and dopamine play crucial roles in mood regulation. When these chemicals are balanced, individuals experience improved emotional stability and overall well-being. Peptide bioregulators work by helping to maintain this balance, providing an avenue for managing mental health more effectively.

Serotonin, often referred to as the "feel-good" neurotransmitter, is essential for maintaining a positive mood. It influences various functions such as appetite, sleep, and emotional state. Low serotonin levels are commonly linked to depression and anxiety. By using peptide bioregulators, it is possible to enhance serotonin production or improve its receptor activity, thus contributing to better mood regulation. For example, peptides can increase the availability of tryptophan, an amino acid precursor to serotonin, which in turn elevates serotonin levels in the brain.

Dopamine, another critical neurotransmitter, is associated with pleasure, motivation, and reward. Imbalances in dopamine levels can lead to feelings of lethargy, lack of motivation, and even depression. Peptide bioregulators can help stabilize dopamine levels by influencing the enzymes that either break down or synthesize dopamine. This stabilization is crucial for maintaining a sense of well-being and motivation, which are vital for daily activities and long-term goals.

Fluctuations in serotonin and dopamine levels can exacerbate symptoms of anxiety and depression. These fluctuations might be triggered by stress, poor nutrition, or genetic factors. Peptide bioregulators offer a potential treatment pathway by modulating these chemical imbalances. Through targeted action, peptides can help maintain a steady flow of neurotransmitters, thereby reducing the mental turmoil caused by sudden drops or spikes in these chemicals. For instance, peptides derived from certain natural sources have been shown to regulate the expression of genes involved in neurotransmitter production, ensuring a more stable emotional state.

Understanding the relationship between peptides and neurotransmitters can empower readers to take control of their mental health. Knowledge is power, and by learning how peptide bioregulators function, individuals can make informed decisions about their mental wellness strategies. This understanding can lead to proactive measures, such as incorporating specific peptides into one's diet or supplement regimen, to maintain mental balance. Empowerment comes from knowing that there are tangible, science-backed tools available for managing mental health.

Research insights provide substantial backing for the use of peptides in balancing neurotransmitter levels. Numerous studies have demonstrated the efficacy of peptide bioregulators in improving mental well-being. For example, research has shown that certain peptides can cross the blood-brain barrier, directly affecting brain chemistry. These peptides interact with receptors specific to serotonin and dopamine, enhancing their signaling pathways. Such findings offer a scientific basis for the claims surrounding peptide bioregulators, making them a credible option for those seeking to improve their mental health.

One noteworthy study involved the administration of neuropeptides to individuals suffering from chronic depression. The results indicated a significant reduction in depressive symptoms, with participants reporting better mood and decreased anxiety levels. Another study focused on the effects of peptides on dopamine regulation in patients with Parkinson's disease, a condition characterized by low dopamine levels. The findings revealed that peptide supplementation led to improved motor functions and emotional stability, highlighting the broader applicability of peptides beyond just mood disorders.

Stress Response Modulation

Peptide bioregulators are emerging as powerful tools in managing the body's stress response, an essential component for emotional stability. This modulation occurs primarily through hormonal adaptation, where these peptides influence stress hormones such as cortisol and adrenaline. In situations that would normally elevate anxiety levels, the presence of peptide bioregulators can help ease these symptoms by ensuring that stress hormones do not spiral out of control.

Hormonal adaptation is crucial during challenging situations. For example, when confronted with a high-pressure work environment or personal life crisis, the body naturally releases stress hormones to prepare for the perceived threat. While this reaction is necessary for survival and coping, prolonged exposure to elevated stress hormones can lead to chronic anxiety. Peptide bioregulators step in by fine-tuning the release and uptake of these hormones, thereby providing a calming effect on the system. This moderation not only helps in reducing immediate anxiety but also prevents the long-term wear and tear on the body that continuous stress can cause.

Maintaining emotional stability is another significant benefit offered by peptide bioregulators. Life often presents stressful events, whether they be unexpected job changes, family issues, or other personal challenges. During these times, keeping one's emotions stable is particularly challenging yet vital. By regulating the body's physiological stress responses, peptide bioregulators contribute to a more balanced emotional state. This regulation acts as a buffer, allowing individuals to navigate through tough periods without experiencing extreme emotional highs and lows.

Enhanced resilience is a key outcome of having a balanced stress response, facilitated by peptide bioregulators. Resilience refers to the ability to recover quickly from difficulties and adapt well to adversity. When the stress response is managed well, it reduces the impact of stressful experiences, enabling quicker recovery and better overall functioning. This increased resilience manifests in daily activities, making it easier to handle routine challenges and bounce back from setbacks. Whether it's maintaining productivity at work, managing relationships, or pursuing personal goals, enhanced resilience improves performance and quality of life.

Scientific research supports the effectiveness of peptide bioregulators in stress response adaptation, adding credibility to their use. Studies have shown that these peptides can positively influence various physiological parameters associated with stress. For instance, a study published in a well-regarded medical journal demonstrated that subjects administered with specific peptide bioregulators exhibited reduced cortisol levels compared to a control group. Additionally, these subjects reported decreased feelings of anxiety and improved mood, underscoring the real-world benefits of peptide supplementation.

Further scientific support comes from animal studies that have examined the underlying mechanisms of how peptide bioregulators function. These studies reveal that peptides can modulate the activity of receptors involved in the stress response, providing a biochemical basis for their effects. For example, experiments on rodents exposed to stressful conditions showed that those treated with peptide bioregulators had a significantly lower stress hormone response compared to untreated counterparts. Such findings pave the way for understanding how these peptides work at a molecular level and support their application in human health.

The role of peptide bioregulators in promoting emotional stability extends beyond individual anecdotes and small-scale studies. Large-scale clinical trials are currently underway to further validate these findings. Preliminary results from these trials indicate that peptide bioregulators could be integrated into mainstream treatment protocols for anxiety and stress-related disorders. Moreover, healthcare practitioners who specialize in mental health and wellness are increasingly recommending peptide supplements to their patients, providing additional layers of professional endorsement.

Reducing Inflammation

Chronic inflammation is a significant factor contributing to various mood disorders, including depression. Emerging evidence suggests that peptide bioregulators can play a crucial role in mitigating this inflammation, thereby reducing symptoms of these mental health conditions. This link between chronic inflammation and mood disorders provides a foundational understanding of how managing inflammation can be a key component in mental wellness strategies.

Depression has long been associated with elevated levels of inflammation in the body. Studies have shown that individuals suffering from chronic inflammatory diseases are at a higher risk of developing depressive symptoms. This connection hints at the potential for peptide bioregulators to intervene by alleviating inflammatory responses. By targeting the root cause—chronic inflammation—peptide bioregulators offer a promising approach to preventing the decline in mood that accompanies many mental health disorders.

Understanding the relationship between inflammation and mood can empower individuals to consider inflammation management as a critical aspect of their mental wellness routine. For example, adopting dietary habits that reduce inflammation or engaging in regular physical exercise known to lower inflammatory markers could complement the use of peptide bioregulators. By incorporating these practices into their daily lives, readers can take proactive steps toward maintaining both their physical and mental health.

The therapeutic potential of peptides in reducing inflammation opens new avenues for mental health treatments. Several peptide bioregulators possess anti-inflammatory properties that can help control the body's immune response. In doing so, they not only alleviate physical symptoms of inflammation but also contribute to enhancing overall emotional stability. This dual benefit makes peptides an intriguing focus for ongoing research and development in mental health interventions.

Clinical studies provide valuable insights into the efficacy of peptides in managing inflammation and improving mental well-being. For instance, research has demonstrated that certain peptides can inhibit pro-inflammatory cytokines, which are proteins involved in the body's inflammatory response. By reducing the levels of these cytokines, peptides can effectively decrease inflammation and its associated negative impact on mood. Such findings underscore the potential of peptides to serve as a natural and effective treatment option for mood disorders linked to inflammation.

In addition to clinical studies, real-world examples further illustrate the benefits of peptides in combating inflammation-related mood disorders. Individuals who have incorporated peptide supplements into their wellness routines often report notable improvements in their mental health, including reduced anxiety and enhanced mood stability. These anecdotal accounts, coupled with scientific research, reinforce the idea that peptides can play a pivotal role in maintaining mental wellness by addressing underlying inflammation.

It's essential to recognize that managing inflammation through peptides represents just one piece of the broader mental health puzzle. However, given the substantial role inflammation plays in mood disorders, integrating peptide bioregulators into a comprehensive mental health strategy holds significant promise. This holistic approach not only targets the physiological aspects of mental health but also supports emotional well-being, offering a well-rounded pathway to improved quality of life.

To effectively utilize peptide bioregulators for inflammation management, it's important for individuals to consult with healthcare professionals. Personalized guidance can ensure that the chosen peptides align with one's specific health needs and conditions. Healthcare providers can offer tailored recommendations and monitor progress, maximizing the therapeutic benefits of peptide supplementation while minimizing any potential risks.

Furthermore, education about the different types of peptide bioregulators and their specific anti-inflammatory effects can enhance readers' understanding and decision-making. For example, peptides like BPC-157 and TB-500 have been studied for their profound anti-inflammatory properties. Knowing the distinct benefits of these peptides can help individuals make informed choices that best suit their mental health goals.

The integration of peptide bioregulators into mental health management requires a balanced approach, combining scientific knowledge with practical application. As the field continues to evolve, ongoing research will likely uncover more precise mechanisms by which peptides influence inflammation and mood, providing even deeper insights into their therapeutic potential. Staying informed about these developments can empower individuals to harness the full benefits of peptide bioregulators in their mental wellness journey.

Improving Mood

Peptide bioregulators have garnered significant attention in recent years for their role in enhancing mood and overall emotional well-being. This section will delve into how these natural compounds can help stabilize mood swings, boost energy levels, improve engagement in self-care activities, and create a positive feedback loop that further amplifies their benefits.

One of the key ways peptide bioregulators influence mood enhancement is through stabilization. Mood swings can be debilitating, making it difficult to maintain a consistent quality of life. Peptide bioregulators have been shown to act on various biochemical pathways that influence mood, thereby helping to even out the highs and lows. For individuals suffering from conditions such as bipolar disorder or chronic stress, this stabilization can be life-changing. By regulating neurotransmitters and other brain chemicals, peptides facilitate a state of balanced emotional health. This stability not only improves day-to-day living but also makes one more resilient to external stressors, promoting a more stable emotional baseline.

In addition to stabilizing mood, peptide bioregulators can significantly boost energy levels. Fatigue and lethargy are common symptoms of depression and other mood disorders. Low energy can make daily tasks feel overwhelming and can perpetuate feelings of sadness and hopelessness. Peptides work by interacting with cellular metabolism, improving the efficiency with which cells produce and utilize energy. This increase in cellular energy translates to better physical and mental stamina. When individuals feel more energized, they are more likely to engage in activities that promote mental health, such as exercise and social interaction, creating a virtuous cycle of well-being.

Improved mood through the use of peptide bioregulators also enhances engagement in wellness activities. Self-care practices, including regular exercise, meditation, and proper nutrition, are essential components of a holistic approach to mental health. However, when someone is struggling with a low mood, finding the motivation to participate in these activities can be challenging. Peptide bioregulators can help by improving overall mood and providing the energy needed to take part in these beneficial activities. For instance, someone who feels more optimistic and energetic is more likely to go for a morning jog or prepare a nutritious meal. Over time, these wellness activities contribute to sustained emotional well-being, thus reinforcing the positive effects of peptides.

Another important aspect of how peptide bioregulators enhance mood is through the creation of a feedback loop. A positive mood makes individuals more receptive to the benefits of peptide bioregulators, thereby amplifying their effectiveness. When mood-improving activities become a regular part of one's routine, the body and mind start to expect and benefit from these enhancements continually. This creates a reinforcing cycle where peptide bioregulators and positive lifestyle choices work together to elevate mood and maintain emotional stability. For example, someone who experiences an initial mood boost from peptides may find it easier to stick to a daily exercise routine. The endorphins released during exercise further elevate their mood, making them more likely to continue using peptides and engaging in other healthy behaviors.

This chapter has provided an in-depth exploration of the role peptide bioregulators play in enhancing mental well-being and emotional stability. By examining how these natural compounds regulate neurotransmitters like serotonin and dopamine, modulate stress responses, and reduce inflammation, we have seen their multifaceted impact on alleviating anxiety and depression. The clinical evidence supporting these benefits highlights the potential of peptide bioregulators as effective tools for improving mood and emotional health.

In understanding the mechanisms through which peptide bioregulators function, individuals are better equipped to make informed decisions about incorporating them into their wellness routines.

These insights pave the way for proactive mental health management, whether through dietary supplements or lifestyle changes. As research continues to uncover more about these potent molecules, their application in mental health strategies is likely to expand, offering new avenues for achieving emotional balance and overall well-being.

CHAPTER 14

Integration into Daily Life

I ntegrating peptide bioregulators into daily routines requires thoughtful planning and attention to detail. As these supplements hold the potential to significantly enhance health outcomes, establishing a consistent method for their intake is crucial. This chapter delves into practical strategies that make it easier to incorporate peptide bioregulators seamlessly into everyday life.

Readers will learn about creating a supplementation schedule that aligns with their lifestyle, optimizing the timing of intake according to personal energy levels and activities, and using technology as an aid for reminders and tracking progress. The chapter also emphasizes the importance of starting slow and gradually building up dosage to ensure the body adapts effectively to the new regimen. By following the methods outlined, individuals can maximize the benefits of peptide bioregulators, ensuring they become a natural part of their health-enhancing routine.

Creating a Supplementation Schedule

Consistency is Key: Establishing a set routine for taking peptide bioregulators can significantly enhance adherence to the regimen. When you follow a consistent schedule, it becomes easier to remember and incorporate this new habit into your daily life. For instance, setting specific times, such as pairing the intake with other daily activities like brushing your teeth or having breakfast, can help ensure that you do not miss a dose. A regular schedule also helps your body adapt to the supplement more effectively, potentially maximizing its benefits.

Each individual can customize their schedule according to their lifestyle, making it more sustainable. Busy professionals might find it convenient to take their supplements during lunch breaks, while athletes might prefer pre- or post-workout slots. Tailoring the timing to fit seamlessly into your existing routine reduces the likelihood of forgetting doses, which can lead to more consistent use and better outcomes.

Living with the Rhythm of Your Body: Aligning peptide bioregulator intake with your personal energy levels or physical activities can optimize results. Every person has a unique circadian rhythm, and understanding these natural cycles can enhance the effectiveness of the supplement. For example, taking peptide bioregulators when you are typically most active could synergize their effects with your body's heightened state of readiness. Similarly, aligning supplementation with periods of rest and recovery, such as before bed, might support repair processes and improve overall well-being.

Listening to your body's signals can also help determine the best times for supplementation. Some individuals may notice they feel more energized after taking peptide bioregulators in the morning, while others might benefit from evening doses that promote relaxation and recovery.

Experimenting with different times of day and observing how your body responds can provide valuable insights into creating an optimal routine.

Utilizing Technology for Reminders: Leveraging apps or alarms can play a crucial role in supporting behavioral changes and maintaining a regimen. With the fast-paced nature of modern life, it is easy to overlook small but important tasks like taking supplements. Technology provides a practical solution by offering customizable reminders that can prompt you at consistent intervals.

There are numerous apps available designed specifically for medication and supplement management. These tools can send notifications to your mobile device, ensuring you never miss a dose. Additionally, some apps allow you to track your intake, monitor any side effects, and even set personalized goals. This structured approach not only aids in consistency but also provides a sense of accomplishment as you stay on track with your health regimen.

Starting Slow: Gradually introducing peptide bioregulators into your routine can mitigate any unexpected reactions. For those new to peptide bioregulators, beginning with a lower dose can help monitor how the body responds before committing to a full regimen. This cautious approach allows you to adjust the dosage and timing as needed, finding what works best for you without overwhelming your system.

Taking things slowly builds confidence in integrating a new health strategy. By starting with smaller amounts, you give your body time to adapt, which can prevent potential discomfort or adverse effects. This gradual introduction also allows you to observe any subtle changes in your health, giving you the opportunity to fine-tune your regimen for optimal benefits.

Consistency is Key

Integrating peptide bioregulators into daily routines is essential for maximizing their benefits and ensuring users achieve their health goals. A structured routine not only enhances the efficacy of these supplements but also improves adherence, making it easier to incorporate them into one's lifestyle.

Establishing a regular timing for taking peptide bioregulators can significantly aid in building lasting habits. Just as the habit of brushing teeth or exercising is cultivated through consistency, supplement intake can become a natural part of daily life. For example, setting a specific time each day for taking peptides—such as first thing in the morning or right before bedtime—can help anchor this activity into one's routine. This scheduled approach ensures that supplementation becomes an automatic behavior rather than something that needs constant mental effort to remember.

Moreover, a consistent routine is crucial for the optimal function of peptide bioregulators within the body. The body thrives on regularity; biological processes such as hormone release, metabolism, and cell regeneration often follow circadian rhythms. By aligning peptide intake with these natural cycles, individuals can enhance the bioavailability and effectiveness of the supplements. Regular consumption allows the body to maintain stable levels of these compounds, thereby supporting continuous physiological regulation.

Customization of the supplementation schedule is another vital aspect of integrating peptide bioregulators into daily life. Each individual has a unique lifestyle, and what works for one person may not be ideal for another. For example, a busy professional might find it more convenient to take supplements during their lunch break, while a fitness enthusiast might prefer to integrate them into a post-workout regimen. Flexibility in timing allows individuals to create a sustainable practice tailored to their daily activities, thus promoting long-term compliance.

Consistency in the use of peptide bioregulators can lead to better absorption and more favorable outcomes. When taken at irregular intervals, the body may not absorb the peptides effectively, reducing their potential benefits. Conversely, regular use helps to prime the body's systems to recognize and utilize these compounds efficiently. Over time, this can translate into enhanced muscle growth for athletes, improved cognitive functions for professionals, and overall wellness for those focused on anti-aging solutions.

Adopting a routine doesn't have to be cumbersome. Simple strategies can be employed to make this process seamless. For instance, linking peptide intake with other established habits—like taking them right after brushing your teeth or before your morning coffee—can make it easier to remember. Creating visual cues or utilizing pill organizers can also assist in keeping the routine intact. These small efforts can significantly improve adherence and make the integration of peptide bioregulators into daily life more manageable.

Understanding personal rhythms and how they align with peptide intake can further optimize the benefits. Recognizing when energy levels are high or when relaxation is needed can guide the timing of supplementation. For instance, some might find that taking peptides in the evening supports better sleep quality, while others might benefit from a morning dose that aligns with peak alertness and activity. Tailoring the schedule in this manner respects the body's natural rhythms and can enhance the effectiveness of the supplements.

In addition, monitoring progress and outcomes regularly is essential to ensure the routine is effective and to make any necessary adjustments. Keeping a simple log or journal where one notes the time of intake and any observed effects can provide valuable insights. Over time, patterns may emerge that indicate the best times for supplementation, allowing for fine-tuning of the schedule. This reflective practice encourages a proactive approach to health management and ensures that the supplementation routine remains aligned with individual goals and responses.

It's worth noting that the journey towards integrating peptide bioregulators into daily life requires patience and persistence. As with any new habit, initial efforts might feel challenging, but consistency will gradually transform these actions into ingrained routines. Celebrating small milestones along the way—such as completing a week of consistent supplementation—can provide motivation and reinforce commitment to the health goals.

Furthermore, seeking support from healthcare providers or nutritionists can offer additional guidance tailored to individual needs. Professionals can provide personalized recommendations based on unique health profiles, helping to optimize the supplementation plan. This collaborative approach ensures that the integration of peptide bioregulators is both safe and effective, enhancing overall well-being.

Living with the Rhythm of Your Body

Understanding how to align your peptide bioregulator intake with personal cycles can maximize benefits and optimize effectiveness. Peptide bioregulators are known for their potential in enhancing performance, recovery, and overall wellness, making it essential to utilize them effectively. One of the most impactful ways to achieve this is by timing the supplementation according to individual routines and bodily responses.

Peptide bioregulators can be particularly beneficial when taken pre- or post-workout. Athletes and fitness enthusiasts often seek quick recovery and improved performance, and these bioregulators can play a crucial role. Taking them before a workout can prepare the body, potentially increasing endurance and strength during exercise. Post-workout intake, on the other hand, aids in faster recovery, helping to repair muscles and reduce soreness. By identifying whether pre- or post-workout supplementation suits you better, you can tailor your approach to enhance your physical activities significantly.

Individuals may find that certain times of the day are more suitable for their peptide bioregulator intake based on unique bodily responses. Some people experience better absorption and effect in the morning when the metabolism is more active, while others might benefit from evening supplementation when the body is winding down. It's important to observe and listen to your body to determine what works best for you. Monitoring how you feel after taking the supplements at different times can offer valuable insights into optimizing your regimen.

Understanding personal cycles is key to determining optimal times for supplementation. Everyone has unique circadian rhythms, which govern various bodily functions such as sleep, energy levels, and hormone production. Aligning your peptide bioregulator intake with these natural cycles can improve their efficacy. For instance, if you notice higher energy levels or better focus at certain times of the day, supplementing during these periods can enhance cognitive benefits and overall well-being. This personalized approach ensures that the supplements work in harmony with your body's natural processes.

Respecting the body's natural rhythms can lead to improved effectiveness of peptide bioregulators. The human body operates on a precise schedule dictated by internal clocks. By synchronizing supplementation with these biological rhythms, you allow the bioregulators to work more efficiently. The body is more receptive to interventions that align with its natural state, leading to better absorption and utilization of the supplements. This synchronized approach not only maximizes the benefits but also minimizes the risk of adverse effects.

To illustrate, consider someone who engages in regular physical activity as part of their daily routine. This individual might experiment with taking peptide bioregulators both before and after workouts to see which timing yields better results. Over time, they might discover that pre-workout supplementation enhances their stamina and muscle performance, while post-workout intake helps with quicker recovery and reduced fatigue. Such observations enable personalized adjustments, ultimately leading to a more effective supplementation strategy.

Additionally, busy professionals concerned about cognitive decline might find that taking peptide bioregulators during their peak mental performance hours could make a significant difference. If these peak hours happen to be in the late morning, a mid-morning dose could support enhanced focus and mental clarity throughout the day. On the other hand, an evening dose might help those who struggle with relaxation and sleep, providing a calming effect that aligns with winding down routines.

Holistic health enthusiasts or individuals exploring alternative medicine options will also appreciate the alignment of supplementation with natural cycles. For example, someone interested in holistic approaches might already practice mindfulness or yoga at specific times of the day. Introducing peptide bioregulators into these routines can create a synergistic effect, enhancing both the physical and mental benefits of their holistic practices. This integration respects and amplifies the body's natural healing processes, promoting a balanced and sustained improvement in health.

Taking the time to understand personal cycles involves self-observation and possibly keeping a journal to track how you feel at different times of the day. Documenting energy levels, mood changes, and physical performance can provide a clear picture of your unique patterns. This information is invaluable for identifying the optimal times for supplementation, ensuring that the peptide bioregulators are working in harmony with your body's rhythms.

In essence, aligning peptide bioregulator intake with personal cycles requires a combination of self-awareness and experimentation. Each person's body responds differently, and what works for one individual might not be as effective for another. However, by paying attention to your body's signals and adjusting your supplementation schedule accordingly, you can significantly enhance the benefits of peptide bioregulators.

Utilizing Technology for Reminders

Technology has revolutionized many aspects of our lives, and when it comes to maintaining a supplementation schedule for peptide bioregulators, digital tools can be incredibly effective. Health enthusiasts, athletes, busy professionals, and those interested in holistic wellness can all benefit from leveraging technology to enhance their health routines.

Digital tools serve as effective reminders, significantly reducing the chance of missed doses. Many people find it challenging to remember taking supplements daily. However, by utilizing smartphone apps or digital calendars, individuals can set up regular notifications that remind them precisely when to take their peptide bioregulators. These timely prompts help integrate the supplementation process seamlessly into everyday life. For instance, simple alarm functions on smartphones can be scheduled to alert users at specific times each day. Some apps are even designed specifically for health and wellness purposes, offering more sophisticated reminder systems that can go beyond basic alarms.

Moreover, engagement with these apps allows individuals to track their intake meticulously. Several apps provide features that let users log each dose they take, ensuring an accurate record is kept over time. Tracking intake helps monitor consistency and adherence to the regimen, which is crucial for realizing the full benefits of peptide bioregulators. Furthermore, these apps often offer functionalities for recording potential side effects or any observable changes in health. Documenting this information can be invaluable for adjusting and optimizing the supplementation program in consultation with healthcare providers.

Personalized notifications make the supplementation regimen feel tailored and less burdensome. Unlike generic reminders, personalized notifications address individual schedules and preferences, promoting a sense of personalization that enhances user engagement. Customization options might include choosing specific tones for alerts, setting reminders based on unique daily patterns, or even motivational messages that encourage adherence to the health plan. This personal touch can transform what might otherwise be a monotonous task into one that feels uniquely suited to the user's lifestyle.

In addition to reminders and tracking, technology aids in creating a structured approach, exponentially increasing success rates. A well-structured regimen is essential for the effectiveness of peptide bioregulators. Technology provides numerous tools to help create and maintain such structure. From calendar integrations that align supplement intake with other daily activities to progress charts that visualize long-term compliance and results, these digital aids offer structure and clarity. Structured approaches improve adherence and help users recognize patterns and correlations between their supplementation and overall well-being. For example, integrating a supplementation schedule into a digital calendar can help balance it alongside work commitments, exercise routines, and social engagements, minimizing disruptions and maximizing consistency.

Starting slow is also recommended, especially for new users adapting to the integration of peptide bioregulators through technological means. Digital platforms can facilitate this gradual introduction by allowing users to set incremental goals and adjust them as they become more comfortable with their regimen. By starting with small, manageable doses and gradually increasing them, users can monitor their body's response and make necessary adjustments without overwhelming themselves. Apps often have features that allow users to modify their schedules and dosage plans on the fly, providing flexibility and control over their health journey.

Adjusting the dosage and timing may be necessary to find an individualized approach that works best. Each person's body responds differently to supplementation, and having the ability to tweak regimens based on real-time data is invaluable. Digital tools enable users to experiment with different dosages and timings, track the outcomes, and refine their approach based on empirical evidence. For instance, if morning doses show better results compared to evening ones, users can adapt their schedules accordingly. This dynamic adjustment capability ensures that the regimen remains efficient and personalized, enhancing its overall effectiveness.

For example, fitness aficionados might find certain apps that cater to their specific needs, offering features like integration with workout schedules or nutritional plans. These specialized apps ensure that peptide bioregulators are taken at optimal times to complement physical training and recovery. Similarly, busy professionals can use productivity apps that incorporate health tracking, allowing them to manage their cognitive health alongside professional tasks efficiently.

Another advantage is the ease of sharing data with healthcare providers. Many apps offer export functions or syncing capabilities with medical records, making it simple for users to share their supplementation history and progress with doctors or nutritionists. This collaboration ensures that the health strategies are backed by professional insights and adjusted as necessary based on monitored outcomes.

Starting Slow

Integrating peptide bioregulators into daily routines can be a game-changer for health enthusiasts, athletes, busy professionals, and individuals interested in holistic health. The benefits of gradually introducing these supplements are manifold, making it a prudent approach for anyone looking to enhance their wellness regimen effectively.

Firstly, one of the primary advantages of gradually integrating peptide bioregulators is the opportunity it provides new users to monitor their body's response. Starting with a lower dosage allows individuals to observe any changes or reactions without the risk of overwhelming their system. This cautious approach helps users identify any initial side effects, such as mild digestive discomfort or temporary changes in energy levels, that could indicate the need for adjustments.

For instance, a health enthusiast might begin with a minimal dose and track their body's reaction over a week. They may find that their energy levels are higher on certain days, or they experience improved sleep quality. These observations are crucial as they provide valuable insights into how the body metabolizes the supplement and whether any modifications are necessary.

In addition to monitoring responses, adjusting the dosage and timing is another critical aspect of gradually introducing peptide bioregulators. Since everyone's physiology is unique, what works for one person might not work for another. By starting slow, users can experiment with different dosages and times of day to find the most effective regimen for their needs.

An athlete, for example, might notice better muscle recovery when taking the supplement post-workout rather than pre-workout. Similarly, a busy professional might find that taking the peptide in the morning enhances mental clarity and focus throughout their demanding workday, while others might benefit from an evening dose that promotes relaxation and better sleep.

This individualized approach not only optimizes the effectiveness of the peptide bioregulators but also builds confidence in this new health strategy. When users see tangible results from their carefully tailored regimen, they are more likely to remain committed to incorporating these supplements into their daily routine. Confidence grows as users become more familiar with how their bodies respond, leading to a more intuitive understanding of their health needs.

Furthermore, gradual introduction prevents overwhelming the body, allowing for better adaptation. Sudden changes in supplementation can stress the body, potentially leading to unwanted side effects which may deter users from continuing with the regimen. A measured approach ensures that the body adjusts slowly and steadily, reducing the risk of adverse reactions and promoting long-term adherence.

Imagine an individual interested in anti-aging solutions who starts with a full dosage right away. They might experience skin breakouts or fatigue, which could discourage them from continuing. However, if they had gradually introduced the peptide bioregulator, their body would have had time to adapt, and they might have avoided these issues altogether.

Journaling the effects experienced during the gradual introduction phase can be immensely beneficial. Keeping a detailed record of physical and mental changes helps users pinpoint precisely when positive shifts occur, correlating them with specific dosages and times. For instance, if a fitness aficionado finds that their endurance improves after two weeks of consistent usage, they can attribute this progress to their careful tracking and incremental adjustments. This process of journaling reinforces the learning experience, providing a clear roadmap for what works best.

Setting goals is another vital guideline when introducing peptide bioregulators slowly. Clear objectives give users something to strive for, keeping motivation high. Whether the goal is improved cognitive function, enhanced athletic performance, or overall well-being, having concrete targets provides direction. Regularly reviewing the progress towards these goals can reinforce the benefits felt, further encouraging consistency and adherence to the supplementation plan.

Regular check-ins with oneself are essential to ensure that the introduction phase is progressing smoothly. Users should routinely evaluate their responses and make adjustments as needed. For example, if an individual notices no significant benefits after a month at a particular dosage, they might decide to increase the amount incrementally. Conversely, if someone experiences unwanted side effects, they might reduce the dosage or adjust the timing. Consistent self-assessment fosters a proactive approach to health, allowing users to fine-tune their regimen for optimal outcomes.

Utilizing assessment tools such as wellness apps or health trackers can complement the process of gradually integrating peptide bioregulators. These tools help users log their intake, note physiological changes, and even remind them to take their supplements consistently. With the aid of technology, individuals can create a structured and efficient approach to their peptide bioregulator regimen, ensuring they stay on track with their health goals.

This chapter has provided easy methods for integrating peptide bioregulators into daily routines, emphasizing the creation of a supplementation schedule and the importance of monitoring progress and outcomes. By establishing a consistent routine, individuals can make taking these supplements a natural part of their day, enhancing adherence and maximizing their benefits. Tailoring the schedule to fit personal lifestyles and aligning intake with natural body rhythms ensures that the supplements work more effectively. Utilizing technology for reminders and starting with smaller doses allows for gradual integration and better adaptation, making the process smoother and more manageable.

Monitoring progress through self-observation, keeping logs, and using digital tracking tools can help refine supplementation schedules further. This reflective practice enables personalized adjustments based on observed outcomes, ensuring the routine remains effective and aligned with individual health goals. By following these strategies, users can seamlessly incorporate peptide bioregulators into their lives, promoting overall wellness, improved performance, and enhanced cognitive function. With patience and persistence, these new habits will become second nature, supporting long-term health and well-being.

CHAPTER 15

Future of Peptide Bioregulator Research

E xploring the future of peptide bioregulator research reveals a promising path toward significant advancements in health and performance enhancement. Peptide bioregulators, small proteins that act at cellular levels, have shown potential to improve numerous biological processes. With ongoing studies, the scope of their applications is expanding, offering new avenues for therapeutic interventions and wellness strategies. From stimulating collagen production for better skin health to boosting muscle growth and recovery in athletes, the possibilities seem limitless. These findings are reshaping our understanding of how targeted peptide usage can optimize both physical and cognitive functions.

In this chapter, we delve into the emerging scientific discoveries surrounding peptide bioregulators and their potential impact on health and wellness. We will explore recent breakthroughs that highlight the unique properties of newly identified peptides and their abilities to influence cell growth, repair, and signaling. The chapter also examines synergistic effects achieved by combining various peptide regimens and investigates long-term benefits of sustained peptide use, such as enhanced cognitive functions. Additionally, we will discuss the integration of genetic testing and advanced peptide synthesis technologies that facilitate personalized healthcare approaches. The implications of these innovations for enhancing athletic performance, improving mental clarity, and supporting holistic health practices will be thoroughly examined, offering readers a comprehensive overview of the exciting future of peptide bioregulator research.

Emerging Scientific Findings

Recent discoveries in peptide bioregulator research have unveiled a plethora of new peptides with unique properties that function at the cellular level to enhance health outcomes. These breakthroughs are illuminating how specific peptides can influence biological processes such as cell growth, repair, and signaling. For instance, some newly identified peptides have been found to effectively stimulate collagen production, which is crucial for skin health and wound healing. This revelation holds great promise for anti-aging solutions and improving overall wellness.

In parallel, ongoing research is exploring the synergistic potential of combining various peptide regimens. By understanding how different peptides interact, scientists are crafting combinations that yield optimized anti-aging and performance-enhancing effects. For example, certain peptide blends are being tested for their ability to both boost muscle growth and improve recovery times in athletes. This dual functionality not only enhances physical performance but also supports long-term health by mitigating risks associated with intense physical activity.

Investigations into the long-term impacts of peptide supplementation are revealing cumulative benefits when these molecules are used over extended periods. Unlike temporary fixes, sustained peptide use appears to provide lasting vitality and improved health markers. For example, studies have shown that consistent peptide intake can lead to enhanced cognitive functions, such as better memory retention and mental clarity. For busy professionals concerned about cognitive decline, these findings are particularly encouraging as they suggest a natural way to maintain mental sharpness.

Moreover, innovations in genetic testing and peptide synthesis are significantly accelerating the pace of discovery and validation in this field. Advanced genetic testing techniques allow researchers to identify individuals who might benefit most from specific peptides based on their genetic makeup. This personalized approach ensures that peptide therapies are tailored to meet individual needs, thus maximizing efficacy. Additionally, rapid advancements in peptide synthesis technology are making it possible to produce complex peptides more efficiently. This efficiency not only reduces costs but also speeds up the availability of new peptide-based treatments.

The implications of these advancements extend beyond mere wellness enhancements. They offer the potential for personalized healthcare approaches that cater to individual needs. For example, through genetic insights, it's becoming feasible to pinpoint specific age-related conditions that could be mitigated or even prevented with targeted peptide interventions. Personalized peptide therapies could revolutionize the management of chronic conditions by providing more effective and tailored treatment options compared to conventional methods.

One guideline for those interested in such personalized approaches is to undergo genetic testing to identify any predispositions to specific health conditions. This step can help determine which peptides would be most beneficial. Consulting with healthcare providers to integrate these findings into a holistic health plan can optimize the benefits of peptide supplementation.

Another significant aspect of recent peptide research is the exploration of their role in enhancing athletic performance. Athletes and fitness enthusiasts are particularly interested in how these bioregulators can naturally boost performance, muscle growth, and recovery times. Current studies indicate that certain peptides can increase the body's natural production of growth hormone, leading to faster muscle development and quicker recovery from strenuous workouts. This natural enhancement offers a safer alternative to synthetic performance enhancers, aligning with the growing preference for holistic and health-conscious fitness strategies.

Furthermore, long-term studies on peptide supplementation highlight a notable decrease in injury rates among athletes who consistently use specific peptides. This benefit stems from improved tissue repair and reduced inflammation, which are critical to maintaining peak physical condition. The sustained vitality observed also correlates with prolonged athletic careers, allowing athletes to perform at high levels for longer periods.

Peptide bioregulators are also gaining attention for their potential cognitive benefits. For busy professionals juggling multiple responsibilities, maintaining cognitive health is paramount. Research indicates that certain peptides can cross the blood-brain barrier and positively affect brain functions. These peptides can enhance neurotransmitter activity, promoting better focus, memory, and mental clarity. For instance, peptides like Cerebrolysin have been studied for their neuroprotective properties, showing promise in preventing cognitive decline and supporting overall brain health.

A recommendation for those seeking to improve cognitive function through peptide supplementation is to begin with peptides known for their neuroprotective effects. Monitoring progress and adjusting dosages under professional supervision can ensure optimal results and safety.

Holistic health enthusiasts are also embracing peptide bioregulators as part of their alternative medicine practices. The natural origins and targeted functionalities of peptides align well with holistic health principles that emphasize balance and preventive care. Peptides offer a non-invasive means to support bodily functions, harmonizing with other natural remedies and lifestyle choices to promote comprehensive well-being.

For individuals integrating peptides into their holistic health regime, it is beneficial to combine them with other natural supplements and practices, such as maintaining a balanced diet, regular exercise, and stress management techniques. This integrated approach can amplify the health benefits derived from peptide use, contributing to overall wellness and longevity.

Potential New Applications

Peptide bioregulators are emerging as powerful tools in the realm of healthcare and wellness. Recent research has highlighted their potential to modulate disease pathways, offering promising new treatment avenues for chronic illnesses. Traditional pharmaceuticals often come with a host of side effects and are not always successful in managing complex diseases. In contrast, peptide bioregulators could offer more targeted therapeutic options. For instance, specific peptides have been shown to interact directly with disease-related proteins, potentially altering the course of illnesses such as diabetes, cardiovascular diseases, and even certain types of cancer. This groundbreaking approach may minimize reliance on pharmaceuticals, offering patients a more precise and less invasive treatment method.

Beyond their role in disease management, peptides are also being studied for their potential to enhance metabolic function and longevity. Emerging studies indicate that certain peptides may play a significant role in weight management and personalized nutrition, two critical areas of interest for health enthusiasts and fitness aficionados alike. By influencing metabolic pathways, these peptides could help regulate appetite, increase energy expenditure, and optimize nutrient absorption. This could lead to more effective strategies for weight loss and maintenance, addressing one of the most persistent challenges in personal health. Moreover, enhanced metabolic function can contribute to improved overall vitality and longevity, aligning well with the goals of anti-aging and wellness communities.

In addition to physical health, researchers are exploring how peptides can influence mood and stress modulation. Mental health conditions like anxiety and depression are becoming increasingly prevalent, and current treatment options often fall short of providing comprehensive relief. Peptides present an innovative avenue for addressing these conditions. For example, some peptides have been found to affect neurotransmitter systems, which play a crucial role in regulating mood and emotional responses. By modulating these systems, peptide-based treatments could offer new hope for individuals struggling with mental health issues. This area of research is particularly exciting because it opens the door to treatments that are not only more effective but also come with fewer side effects compared to traditional psychiatric medications.

Another promising application of peptide bioregulators lies in the field of dermatology. Scientific advancements suggest that peptides may significantly improve skin health through innovative formulations. The cosmetic industry is already taking notice, with many skincare products now featuring peptides as key ingredients. These peptides work by stimulating collagen production, enhancing skin elasticity, and promoting cellular repair. As a result, they can help reduce signs of aging, such as wrinkles and fine lines, providing a more youthful appearance. Additionally, peptides can improve skin barrier function, which is essential for maintaining hydration and protecting against environmental damage. By incorporating peptide bioregulators into skincare routines, individuals can achieve both aesthetic and wellness benefits.

The potential applications of peptide bioregulators extend far beyond their current uses, encouraging us to consider future possibilities. One of the most exciting aspects of peptide research is its multidisciplinary nature. Combining expertise from various fields, including biology, chemistry, and medicine, can lead to groundbreaking discoveries and innovations. For instance, interdisciplinary collaboration could pave the way for more refined and effective peptide-based therapies, optimizing their impact on health and performance.

As we look ahead, the integration of peptide bioregulators into mainstream healthcare and wellness practices seems increasingly likely. Ongoing research will undoubtedly continue to unlock new applications and refine existing ones, making peptide bioregulators a cornerstone of modern medicine and personal health. Whether it's through their potential to revolutionize disease treatment, enhance metabolic function, improve mental health, or boost skin vitality, peptides hold the promise of a healthier, more vibrant future.

It's essential for health enthusiasts, athletes, busy professionals, and anyone interested in holistic health approaches to stay informed about these advancements. By understanding the current state and future potential of peptide bioregulator research, individuals can make more informed decisions about their health and wellness strategies. This knowledge empowers them to explore new frontiers in personal health, leveraging the latest scientific breakthroughs to enhance their quality of life.

Technological Advancements in Research

Advancements in technology are rapidly transforming the field of peptide bioregulator research. One of the most significant breakthroughs is the innovation in genetic testing and peptide synthesis, which have dramatically enhanced the speed and accuracy of peptide discovery and validation processes. Genetic testing allows researchers to identify specific gene expressions linked to health conditions, enabling them to pinpoint corresponding peptides that can target these expressions for therapeutic interventions. This precision not only shortens the time required for discovering new peptides but also improves the reliability of the findings, ensuring that they can be more effectively applied in clinical settings.

Peptide synthesis has also seen remarkable improvements, particularly through automation and high-throughput screening techniques. These advancements enable scientists to create a vast array of peptide sequences quickly and efficiently, facilitating the exploration of their biological activity and therapeutic potential. Traditional methods of peptide synthesis were labor-intensive and prone to errors, but with modern automated systems, researchers can now generate large libraries of peptides and test them against various biological targets in a fraction of the time previously required. This accelerated pace of discovery is crucial for developing new peptide-based therapies that can enhance health and performance.

Advanced imaging techniques play a pivotal role in understanding peptide interactions at a molecular level. Technologies such as cryo-electron microscopy (cryo-EM) and single-molecule fluorescence resonance energy transfer (smFRET) allow scientists to visualize peptides within their biological environments with astonishing detail. Cryo-EM, for instance, enables the visualization of complex biomolecular structures at near-atomic resolution, providing insights into how peptides interact with proteins and other cellular components. Understanding these interactions is essential for elucidating the mechanisms through which peptides exert their biological effects and for designing peptides with optimized therapeutic properties.

Similarly, smFRET allows researchers to monitor the dynamic behavior of individual peptide molecules in real-time. By labeling peptides with fluorescent probes and observing their interactions under a microscope, scientists can gain a deeper understanding of how peptides bind to their targets, undergo conformational changes, and initiate signaling pathways. These advanced imaging techniques offer a window into the intricate world of peptide biology, revealing details that were previously hidden from view and guiding the development of more effective and targeted peptide-based treatments.

Data analytics and machine learning tools are revolutionizing the way researchers predict peptide behavior and optimize therapeutic approaches. The sheer volume of data generated by modern peptide research can be overwhelming, but advanced computational tools can analyze this data to identify patterns and make predictions about peptide activity. Machine learning algorithms, in particular, excel at processing large datasets and uncovering relationships that might not be immediately apparent. By training algorithms on known peptide sequences and their biological effects, researchers can develop models that predict the efficacy and safety of newly synthesized peptides, streamlining the drug development process.

These predictive models are invaluable for optimizing therapeutic approaches. For example, by analyzing the structure-activity relationships of peptides, machine learning can suggest modifications to enhance their stability, bioavailability, or target specificity. This ensures that the peptides developed are not only effective but also practical for clinical use. Data analytics also facilitate personalized medicine approaches, where treatment regimens can be tailored to the genetic and biological profiles of individual patients, maximizing the benefits of peptide-based therapies while minimizing potential side effects.

Technological advancements are also fostering interdisciplinary collaboration, which is vital for translating research findings into clinical practice. The complexity of peptide bioregulator research necessitates input from multiple scientific disciplines, including biology, chemistry, pharmacology, and bioinformatics. Advances in communication technologies and collaborative platforms are making it easier for researchers from different fields to work together, share data, and integrate their expertise. This collaborative approach accelerates the translation of basic research into practical applications, ensuring that promising peptide discoveries move swiftly from the laboratory bench to the bedside.

For instance, biologists studying the physiological effects of peptides can collaborate with chemists who specialize in synthesizing novel peptide sequences. Pharmacologists can then evaluate the therapeutic potential of these peptides in preclinical models, while bioinformaticians apply data analytics to refine the formulations and predict clinical outcomes. This interconnected workflow not only enhances the efficiency of the research process but also ensures that the resulting therapies are grounded in a comprehensive understanding of peptide biology and pharmacology.

Furthermore, the integration of technological advancements into the clinical trial process is streamlining the development of peptide-based therapies. Electronic data capture systems, remote monitoring tools, and decentralized trial designs are improving the efficiency and accuracy of clinical research. These innovations reduce the administrative burden on researchers, allow for real-time data collection, and make it easier to recruit and retain study participants. As a result, clinical trials can be conducted more swiftly and with greater precision, accelerating the approval and commercialization of new peptide therapies.

Interdisciplinary Collaboration

Interdisciplinary collaboration plays a pivotal role in the advancement of peptide bioregulator research. By bringing together expertise from various fields, comprehensive and innovative solutions can be developed to address complex health challenges.

Firstly, the synergy between biologists, chemists, and medical professionals is crucial for the thorough investigation and innovation of peptide bioregulators. Biologists contribute their deep understanding of cellular processes and organismal biology, which is essential for identifying and characterizing new peptides. Chemists, on the other hand, bring their expertise in molecular synthesis and structural analysis, enabling the design and production of peptide molecules with specific desired properties. Medical professionals provide invaluable insights into clinical applications and patient care, ensuring that the developed peptides are not only effective but also safe for human use. This triad of expertise creates a robust framework for comprehensive peptide research that spans from basic scientific discovery to applied therapeutic solutions.

Moreover, interdisciplinary collaboration is fundamental in developing personalized healthcare solutions based on peptide bioregulator data. Personalized medicine aims to tailor medical treatment to the individual characteristics of each patient, and peptide bioregulators hold great potential in this field due to their specific actions at the molecular level. By integrating knowledge from genomics, proteomics, and clinical practice, researchers can develop peptide-based therapies that are customized to the genetic and biochemical profiles of individuals. For instance, certain peptides may be more effective in individuals with specific genetic mutations or metabolic conditions, leading to more targeted and efficient treatments. Such personalized approaches have the potential to significantly enhance health outcomes and minimize adverse effects, paving the way for more precise and individualized medical care.

The integration of bioinformatics and computational biology is another critical aspect of interdisciplinary efforts in peptide research. The complexity of peptide interactions within biological systems requires sophisticated tools for data analysis and interpretation. Bioinformatics provides the necessary computational methods to manage and analyze large datasets, such as those generated by high-throughput sequencing and proteomics studies. Computational biology, meanwhile, uses mathematical modeling and simulations to predict the behavior of peptides in different physiological contexts. These disciplines enable researchers to decipher the intricate networks of peptide interactions, identify potential therapeutic targets, and optimize peptide design. For example, machine learning algorithms can be used to predict the stability and efficacy of novel peptides, thereby accelerating the development process. The enhanced ability to analyze complex peptide data through bioinformatics and computational biology is thus a key driver of innovation in this field.

Partnerships with pharmaceutical companies and biotech firms are essential for translating peptide research into practical applications. While academic and research institutions often focus on the initial stages of discovery and validation, the commercialization of peptide-based therapies requires additional resources and expertise that industry partners can provide. Pharmaceutical companies have the infrastructure and regulatory experience necessary to conduct large-scale clinical trials, manufacture peptide drugs in compliance with stringent quality standards, and navigate the approval process with regulatory agencies. Biotech firms, on the other hand, are agile and innovative, capable of rapidly developing and testing new peptide formulations and delivery methods. Collaborative efforts between these entities facilitate the seamless transition from lab bench to bedside, ensuring that groundbreaking discoveries in peptide bioregulators reach patients efficiently and effectively.

Furthermore, the practical application of peptide research benefits greatly from interdisciplinary collaboration. Beyond the scientific and technical aspects, successful implementation also involves considerations related to market demand, economic feasibility, and ethical implications. Interdisciplinary teams that include experts in public health, economics, and ethics can address these broader issues, ensuring that peptide-based therapies are not only scientifically sound but also socially responsible and economically viable. For example, public health experts can assess the potential impact of new peptide treatments on population health, while economists can evaluate cost-effectiveness and accessibility. Ethicists, meanwhile, ensure that the development and distribution of peptide therapies adhere to ethical principles, safeguarding patient rights and promoting equitable access.

Ethical and Regulatory Considerations

In the rapidly advancing field of peptide bioregulator research, ethical and regulatory aspects are critical to ensure the responsible development and application of these promising compounds. Ethical considerations in this context are paramount, particularly when it comes to ensuring informed consent and patient safety during clinical trials.

Informed consent is a fundamental ethical requirement. It involves providing potential participants with all necessary information about the study's purpose, procedures, risks, and benefits, enabling them to make an educated decision about their involvement. Researchers must ensure that participants understand what they are consenting to, using clear and comprehensible language. This goes beyond merely obtaining a signature; it means fostering a truly informed decision-making process. Furthermore, ongoing communication is essential, as new information may emerge during the study that could impact participants' willingness to continue.

Patient safety is another crucial ethical consideration. Clinical trials involving peptide bioregulators must prioritize minimizing harm and maximizing the potential for benefit. This includes rigorous preclinical testing, continuous monitoring of participants, and promptly addressing any adverse effects that arise. Additionally, researchers should design studies to mitigate risks, ensuring that trial protocols are scientifically sound and ethically justified.

The rapid advancements in peptide research necessitate adaptable and forward-thinking regulatory frameworks. Current regulations may not adequately address the unique challenges posed by peptide bioregulators, which operate through novel mechanisms of action and offer unprecedented therapeutic potential. Regulators must work closely with researchers to develop clear guidelines that ensure the safe usage and distribution of peptide-based therapies.

One approach to achieving this is by establishing specialized committees or advisory boards composed of experts in peptide research, ethics, and regulatory affairs. These bodies could review and update guidelines regularly, taking into account the latest scientific developments and ethical considerations. Moreover, international cooperation is essential, as peptide research often spans multiple countries. Harmonizing regulatory standards across borders can facilitate global collaboration and streamline the approval process for new peptide therapies.

Transparency in addressing potential risks and benefits is vital for gaining public trust and acceptance of peptide-based therapies. Both researchers and regulators must communicate openly about the limitations and uncertainties associated with these treatments. This involves being honest about the current state of knowledge, acknowledging unknowns, and clearly outlining the potential benefits versus the risks.

For instance, while peptide bioregulators hold great promise for enhancing health and performance, their long-term effects are not yet fully understood. Public disclosures should include information on known side effects, the expected duration of benefits, and any ongoing research aimed at answering unresolved questions. Engaging in transparent dialogue helps manage expectations and fosters a sense of shared responsibility among all stakeholders.

Ongoing dialogue between researchers, policymakers, and the public is crucial for balancing innovation with ethical responsibility. Peptide bioregulators represent a new frontier in medicine, and navigating this landscape requires input from diverse perspectives. By fostering open communication channels, stakeholders can collaboratively address ethical dilemmas, regulatory challenges, and public concerns.

Regular public forums, stakeholder meetings, and advisory panels can serve as platforms for such dialogue. These gatherings provide opportunities for scientists to explain their work, answer questions, and listen to feedback from the community. Policymakers can use these insights to shape regulations that protect public health while supporting scientific progress. In turn, the public gains a better understanding of peptide bioregulators, which can lead to more informed opinions and decisions regarding these therapies.

Ethical and regulatory considerations in peptide bioregulator research also extend to issues of accessibility and equity. Ensuring that the benefits of these therapies are available to a broad population, rather than just a privileged few, is a significant ethical concern. Strategies to address this might include implementing fair pricing models, supporting policies that promote equitable access, and conducting research that considers diverse populations.

Equity in clinical trials is also important. Diverse participant pools enhance the generalizability of findings and help identify variations in treatment efficacy and safety among different demographic groups. Researchers should strive to recruit participants from various backgrounds, including different ages, genders, ethnicities, and socioeconomic statuses. This ensures that the resulting therapies are safe and effective for all segments of the population.

Another key ethical issue is the potential use of peptide bioregulators for human enhancement. While these compounds have the potential to improve health and treat diseases, they might also be used to enhance normal functions, such as cognitive abilities or physical performance. This raises questions about fairness, consent, and the societal implications of widespread enhancement.

Regulations must carefully delineate between therapeutic and enhancement uses of peptides, ensuring that ethical principles guide their application. Public discussions and policy debates are essential to determine acceptable boundaries and societal norms regarding enhancement. Engaging bioethicists, sociologists, and other experts can provide valuable insights into the broader implications of peptide use, helping to craft thoughtful and balanced policies.

In this chapter, we delved into the promising future of peptide bioregulators and how ongoing research is uncovering their potential to enhance health and performance. We explored various peptides and their unique roles in supporting cellular functions like growth, repair, and signaling. By examining their impact on skin health, muscle growth, and cognitive function, we highlighted the broad spectrum of benefits these molecules offer. Furthermore, we discussed the importance of personalized peptide therapies based on genetic makeup, which can optimize individual health outcomes.

The chapter also emphasized the technological advancements accelerating peptide research, such as genetic testing and sophisticated synthesis methods. These innovations enable a quicker and more precise discovery of new peptides, enhancing their therapeutic applications. For athletes, busy professionals, and holistic health enthusiasts alike, understanding these advancements provides valuable insights into how peptide bioregulators can be integrated into wellness strategies to support longevity and overall vitality.

CONCLUSION

I n our journey through the fascinating world of peptide bioregulators, we have uncovered their incredible potential to transform various aspects of our health and wellness. These small but mighty molecules have demonstrated profound benefits, ranging from anti-aging properties that rejuvenate our cells and tissues to performance boosts that athletes can harness to achieve peak physical condition. This isn't mere speculation; the scientific community is increasingly recognizing and validating the substantial impact of peptide bioregulators.

For health enthusiasts seeking youthful vitality, peptide bioregulators offer hope beyond traditional methods. They work at a cellular level, promoting repair and regeneration, which helps counteract the inevitable march of time. The practical benefits for athletes are equally impressive. By integrating peptide bioregulators into their regimes, they can enhance muscle growth, improve recovery times, and protect against injury, allowing for sustained high-performance levels. Busy professionals, too, stand to gain immensely from these findings. Cognitive decline, memory lapses, and loss of focus can hinder productivity, but peptide bioregulators provide a way to safeguard mental clarity and sharpen cognitive functions.

The importance of translating these theoretical insights into daily practice cannot be overstated. Embracing the practical applications of peptide bioregulators can seem daunting at first glance, but it need not be so. As discussed in earlier chapters, there are straightforward ways to incorporate these peptides into your regimen. From oral supplements that can easily fit into your morning routine to topical applications that seamlessly integrate into your existing skincare habits, the means to leverage these powerful agents are readily accessible. It's about taking small, intentional steps towards incorporating these tools into your life for tangible, long-term benefits.

Moreover, the benefits of peptide bioregulators aren't confined to isolated areas of health. They represent a holistic approach to wellness, impacting everything from physical strength and endurance to mental acuity and emotional well-being. We are on the cusp of a new understanding of how our bodies function and heal, and peptide bioregulators are at the forefront of this paradigm shift. This book has aimed to equip you with knowledge and strategies to harness this potential effectively.

As exciting as the current landscape is, the realm of peptide bioregulator research is ever-evolving. The scientific advancements we have explored merely scratch the surface of what is possible. Continuous research promises to unlock even more applications and benefits, making it an exhilarating field to follow. I encourage you, dear reader, to remain curious and engaged. Keep abreast of the latest findings, seek out reputable sources of information, and perhaps even participate in ongoing studies if opportunities arise.

Your journey into understanding peptide bioregulators is just beginning. Think of this as a lifelong adventure into health and wellness, where each new discovery enhances your quality of life. The path you are now on will not only benefit you but could also inspire and inform others within your circles who are searching for effective, science-backed solutions for their health concerns.

Now that you possess this powerful knowledge, the next step is action. Imagine waking up each day feeling renewed, invigorated, and ready to tackle whatever comes your way. By incorporating peptide bioregulators into your daily life, you can actively take control of your health and experience a profound transformation. This is not an unreachable dream but a realistic goal that starts with a single, simple step. Whether it's deciding to try a recommended supplement, adjusting your skincare routine, or making informed dietary changes, each action brings you closer to a healthier, more vibrant you.

Success stories abound of individuals who've taken that first step and witnessed remarkable improvements in their well-being. Their experiences serve as testaments to the efficacy of peptide bioregulators and as inspiration for your own journey. You're standing at the threshold of significant positive change, and all it requires is your willingness to move forward. Take that step today—embrace the promise of peptide bioregulators and become an active participant in your own health revolution.

Remember, transforming your health isn't about radical overhauls but about consistent, deliberate actions that accumulate over time. Every small effort contributes to a larger picture of enhanced vitality and longevity. Start with manageable increments—perhaps incorporating a single peptide supplement or modifying one aspect of your diet—and gradually build upon these foundations. The cumulative effect will be a noticeable improvement in your overall health and well-being.

In conclusion, the exploration of peptide bioregulators opens up a world brimming with possibilities. It offers practical, scientifically backed solutions to enhance physical performance, slow down aging processes, boost cognitive functions, and promote holistic health. You've been equipped with the knowledge; now it's time to put it into practice. Let this be the beginning of your commitment to better health—one that empowers you, enriches your life, and sets a shining example for those around you. Take charge of your wellness journey today, and relish the transformative power of peptide bioregulators.

FREE SUPPLEMENTARY RESOURCES

Are you interested in unlocking the secrets to prolonged youth and enhanced performance? Our book, *"The Peptide Bioregulator Revolution"*, provides you with comprehensive insights into cutting-edge advancements in peptide bioregulation that promote anti-aging, muscle growth, and cognitive enhancement.

But there's more! To further boost your journey towards achieving youthful vitality and peak performance, we're offering an exclusive bonus resource available for download—completely free. Don't miss this opportunity to expand your knowledge and apply groundbreaking strategies to maintain optimal health and vitality well into your later years!

Use QR code to claim your bonus:

Download Your Bonus!

Best regards,

Matthew Clarke-Hunter

13553939R00070